To all the athletes who have taught us so much over the years.

CONTENTS

FOREWORDS

In 2009, I had the great opportunity to run personal bests in the marathon (2:09:15) and the half marathon (1:01:00). My personal best in the marathon came at the 2009 New York City Marathon, where I was the first American to win the race since Alberto Salazar in 1982. Such performances are welcome news not only because I am running my best times well into my professional career, which consists of an Olympic medal, American records, and 18 USA Track and Field championships, but also because they are coming after the worst injury I have ever had. In November 2007, I suffered a pelvis fracture during the U.S. Olympic Marathon Trials. Although this injury most likely occurred during the race, I continued to run and finished the marathon. Despite the extreme pain and discomfort, I initially didn't recognize that the injury was as severe as it was. I knew I had pushed my body and overcompensated for my cramped calves in order to finish the race. As a result I didn't get an MRI immediately, and it was Dr. Lewis Maharam who insisted on a very specific MRI in order to diagnose the problem. Once the correct diagnosis was made, my rehabilitation process was structured and focused. The road back from that potentially career-ending injury to running personal bests has been a tremendous test of my faith and determination. Many people deserve credit for helping me make this comeback, and it would take some time to explain all of the people involved. But without a doubt, one of the key contributors to my comeback has been Dr. Krista Austin.

Interestingly, I first met Krista while taking an ice bath at the San Diego Olympic Training Center in 1999. At that time, I was a recently turned professional athlete, and Krista was a master's student at San Diego State University and an intern at the Olympic Training Center. We struck up a conversation, and 10 years later not only are we good friends but I consider Krista a key component of Team Meb as well. I truly believe that everything happens for a reason and that God puts people in our lives for a reason. When I first met Krista in San Diego, I could not imagine the impact she would have on my life.

For years I have consulted with Krista about my athletic potential and how to go about realizing it. Krista's scientific knowledge and expertise allow her to analyze what a specific athlete's body can and cannot do and how an athlete can maximize his or her athletic potential. I cannot begin to convey just how highly I respect Krista for her superior knowledge in the fields of exercise physiology and nutrition. Krista communicates information directly to me and also shares her insight with my long-time coach Bob Larsen. Krista also advises my wife, Yordanos Asgedom, on the best type of meals for me based on type of training and competition schedule. Finally, in this day and age of drug cheats, I trust Krista to recommend vitamins to supplement my diet. I do not take any supplement without the prior consent and consultation of Dr. Krista Austin. I hope it is sufficient to say that Krista knows her stuff, and I trust her with this very important component of my athletic career.

Krista has earned my trust not only through the expertise in her field but also because of her unique ability and desire to help me and other world-class athletes be the best we can be. Krista has supported me through the ups and downs of my athletic career. She would come visit me and my family in Mammoth and has opened her home in Colorado Springs to me and my family. Krista is such an important person in my life that my three-year-old daughter calls her "Auntie Krista."

After my injury during the U.S. Olympic Marathon Trials, I worked with many doctors throughout the different stages of my rehabilitation. Throughout every step of the way, Krista was there to consult with me and refer me to different specialists. In September 2008, almost one year after my injury, Krista helped coordinate the most intensive part of my rehabilitation. She invited me to the Olympic Training Center in Colorado Springs in order to continue my altitude training and simultaneously rehab to get my body stronger. What was meant to be a one-week visit turned out to be a two-month intensive rehabilitation and training period.

I learned many things during the almost year-long rehabilitation process. First, an athlete must work harder and must be more dedicated when injured than when healthy. Second, having a strong support group during this time is more important than having unlimited supporters when all is going well. During my recovery process, Krista exemplified the meaning of a friend and professional. As a friend, Krista hosted me in her home and then opened her home to my wife and two kids so I could continue with the productive process and not have to be separated from my beloved family for so long. As a professional, Krista helped arrange for me to take advantage of all the resources available through the U.S. Olympic Committee. During this time, Krista's consultation about the recovery process and my future outlook played a key role in preparing my mind and body for what it is doing today—running better than ever. I am very fortunate to count Dr. Krista Austin as a good friend and key advisor. I am also very glad she is able to share her amazing insight with you. Pay attention; Dr. Austin knows her stuff!

Mebrahtom "Meb" Keflezighi
Olympic silver medalist

I first met Bob in 2002. We were at an open-water swim lake in Colorado, just chatting about triathlon, and I discovered he was a sports nutritionist. I was attempting my first Ironman that year and needed some guidance on the nutrition for that event, and Bob offered to help me out. It turns out that Bob not only is an expert in this field but also has a wealth of knowledge in many other areas of endurance training. I enjoyed all our conversations, learning so much and wanting to talk for hours.

Although my humbling results at Hawaii Ironman (19th overall) led me back to the path of my Olympic Team pursuit, my nutrition there was perfect. I continued working with Bob on other aspects of my training through 2003 in my preparation for the 2004 Olympic Triathlon Trials. His guidance and advice contributed greatly to my ultimate success in that venture and beyond. In 2008, Bob helped me prepare for a winning performance at the Leadville 100-mile (160 km) mountain bike race. And in 2009 we joined coaching forces to create Elite Multisport Coaching, a triathlon community that works with youth and elite athletes of all disciplines and abilities.

Bob's first book, *Nutrition Periodization for Endurance Athletes*, really led athletes, coaches, and sports nutritionists to think outside the box. And since that book was published, Bob continues to push the envelope of sports nutrition, going beyond the traditional views of what to eat to focus on how to use our diets to optimize our performance and our well-being throughout the year. I think athletes of all abilities will benefit greatly from reading this new book.

Susan Williams
2004 Olympic triathlon bronze medalist

PREFACE

The first question we often ask athletes when they enter our office is out of 100 percent, how much does nutrition affect their performance? Typically, most athletes are kind enough to give nutrition about 10 to 15 percent and attribute the rest to training and recovery. This response tells us a great deal about how these athletes are viewing their food. When we point out that an athlete's nutrition should be designed to support training and enhance recovery, athletes realize that nutrition can affect performance 100 percent.

Timing nutrient ingestion is a concept that has become increasingly popular in the world of sport performance. When the primary goal between training sessions is to recover, nutrition becomes a key component that will allow the body to adapt to the imposed training demand; thus nutrition to support the recovery process and adaptations to training must start before training even begins. This concept might best be understood by viewing the body as a furnace and its energy supply as the fuel for the furnace. The furnace in a house functions best when we ensure that enough fuel is readily available, and a steady supply of fuel to the furnace keeps it functioning most efficiently. The furnace also runs best when we consider the type of fuel we use to maintain the fire. A high-quality fuel will ensure that the furnace runs most effectively, whereas low-quality fuel can lead to eventual breakdown of the system. In the same sense, if an athlete does not fuel the body at regular intervals throughout the day and provides the body with poor food choices for the energy demand it is under (i.e., training load), then recovery from training cannot occur and adaptation cannot take place. The furnace is equal to the engine of the human body, which is also known as metabolism. The rate of metabolism is dependent on consistently needing to operate the body within an optimal range. If the body is deprived of food, metabolism is reduced to compensate, and over time the body will operate continuously under this reduced rate. When quality food such as whole grains, fruits, and protein is provided steadily throughout the day, metabolism increases and thus helps minimize fat stores while improving muscle mass.

The timing, type, and volume of carbohydrate, protein, and fat consumed throughout the day are critical for restoring overall muscle function and body homeostasis. Several decades of scientific research has shown us that centering an athlete's food and fluid consumption around exercise (before, during, and after) can significantly help support the demands of sport training. The greatest evidence for timing nutrient ingestion initially came from studies examining the effects of timing carbohydrate ingestion. These studies showed that muscle glycogen (carbohydrate stored within the muscle) was restored faster when athletes were fed carbohydrate within the first hour after exercise than when the intake was delayed. Since this time, a number of studies have emerged to show that timing nutrient ingestion can promote enhanced recovery from training, create positive training adaptations, improve body composition, support immune health, and thus enhance performance.

Athletes come in all body shapes and sizes, and all have personal sport performance goals. However, with these goals come a variety of different genetics, training backgrounds, eating habits, and personal histories that make each athlete's needs unique—even within the same sport or family. As a result, timing nutrient ingestion must take into account the athlete's own instinctive eating, environment, food preferences, and psychological view of food. To properly apply the concept of timing nutrient ingestion, it must be realized that *we eat to train rather than train so we can eat*. For many, this may be a new way of thinking about nutrition, and an open mind-set that is ready to consider new ideas is necessary in order to adopt the principles that are presented. Our goal in this book is to provide the athlete, coach, and support staff a knowledge base and toolbox that will allow them to develop their own nutrition programs that are geared to optimize adaptations to training and enhance recovery from training.

In the first chapter, we familiarize you with the basis and background we believe is necessary to lay the foundation for timing nutrient ingestion. From there, we give you the knowledge behind the methods so that you have a full understanding of how and why timing nutrient ingestion works. Toward the end of the book, we combine that knowledge and personal preferences to bring all of this together for an optimal performance nutrition plan.

Note for Weight-Classified Athletes

Over the years, my focus on how to work with athletes in weight-classified sports has significantly changed. I used to frown upon athletes who appeared to cut large amounts of weight going into competition (yet won). Instead, I followed the conservative approach to getting an athlete to make weight, allowing only a 2 to 3 percent body-weight cut in the days leading up to competition. Losing weight through a breakdown in muscle mass was taboo, and the thought of even assisting in a sauna-based weight cut was never even a question. I was mainly influenced by a lack of knowledge regarding the sport and the science.

The change in my mentality happened over the past several years. I met brothers who shared the goal to become world and Olympic champions, and based on height and body size they should have competed in the same weight category. The option to go up an additional weight class and gain mass was not there, nor was it healthy for them to sit 2 to 3 percent out from their weight class—they most likely would never have been successful. In the end, one sibling would have to sacrifice for the other if they were both to compete, and they would do it—with or without me. Today, they stand and compete as world champions, and Olympic medals hang around their necks, and I have become a better scientist and practitioner for it.

Throughout this book, I have intentionally addressed weight-classified sports and the upper limits of weight cutting. It is important that athletes, parents, and coaches consider the age and stage of development; any form of weight cutting should be minimized in young athletes who are still growing. Every athlete is different, and the goal is to achieve the best performance in the safest manner possible. Although guidelines are provided in this book, I hope that you seek assistance in working with a physiologist who knows your sport and can help optimize this lifelong process.

Please be safe,
Krista Austin

ACKNOWLEDGMENTS

I would like to thank some of the many mentors, coaches, and other influential people who helped make this book a unique combination of science and real-life experience. Thanks to my mentors Michael Buono, Fred Kolkhorst, Mike Shannon, and Emily Haymes for giving me the freedom to experiment and learn in an open environment while at the same time challenging me to become the scientist and practitioner that I am today. Many thanks also to Melinda Manore for her energy, openness, and insight into the field of sports nutrition.

An enormous thanks to the elite coaches who have influenced and believed in me over the years: George Dallam, JJ Clark, Blackman Ihem, Joe Vigil, Paul Ratcliffe, Jean Lopez, Bill Sweetenham, Kevin Renshaw, Jorg Gotz, Per Nilsson, and Zeke Jones. My work with these coaches' athletes has made this book possible. Thanks to all the athletes who were willing to try a new point of view and have kept the fire burning by giving me new challenges at every turn.

Finally, thanks to my parents, Steve and Gail, and to my friends and colleagues Bo, Mike, Jon, Meredith, Keri, Sunde, and William for always supporting me. Last and definitely not least, thanks to Auntie's little angel, Sara, who sat by my side on many nights as I wrote this book and reminded me of what is important in life.

Krista Austin

Many people throughout my career have been influential, but most notable is my first graduate advisor, Dr. Matt Hickey, who taught me not only how to review research with a critical eye but also to have an open mind when approaching research and its application to sport. This has allowed me to blend science into real-life application, which is seen throughout this book. Both critical thinking and outside-the-box thinking have enabled me to apply complex principles of sports nutrition to athletes and coaches in a user-friendly manner.

Additionally, I would like to extend thanks to my family for all of their support throughout the countless hours of "research" I spent in my own physical training, which allowed me to put my tough questions to the test in real-life training situations. Being in the trenches as an athlete allows me to fine-tune the nutrition concepts that science provides.

Bob Seebohar

Principles of Nutrient Timing

Performance nutrition is about strategically utilizing the food an athlete consumes to gain an advantage in training adaptations and performance. Through the use of nutrient timing, food can be used to enhance the energy systems, improve body composition, and increase stamina for improved performance. Nutrient timing is designed to use physiological principles to drive what type of foods athletes eat and when they eat them. Using these principles puts the body in an optimal state for training and competition.

Physiological Basis for Nutrient Timing

Several lines of scientific evidence provide the basis for timing nutrient ingestion. The body's response to exercise in terms of hormone control and muscle function and its response to different types of carbohydrate and protein create the foundation for understanding how timing nutrition specifically to the muscles' functional needs is optimal for an athlete. Together, these responses produce the greatest evidence, which is the effect on body composition, glycogen stores, protein balance, and rehydration.

Hormonal Control

Hormonal responses to exercise are dependent on training intensity, training duration, training volume, and the fitness level of the person. The key **hormones** involved in the regulation of muscle function are epinephrine, norepinephrine, insulin, cortisol, and glucagon. Figure 1.1 shows how these hormone levels change with increasing exercise duration. The hormones epinephrine and norepinephrine are called **neurotransmitters** and are responsible for stimulating the breakdown of stored fat and **glycogen** for use as energy during exercise. With the onset of exercise, epinephrine and norepinephrine rapidly increase.

Insulin is the hormone responsible for the integration of fuel metabolism at rest and during exercise. The levels of insulin determine how much of the body's needed energy will be derived from the breakdown of fat, carbohydrate, and protein. When an athlete is in a fasted state, less insulin is produced, and fats and proteins are recruited to provide fuel for the body. With food consumption, insulin levels increase so that consumed carbohydrate, fat, and protein can be utilized for fuel or stored by

hormone – A substance that is produced in one of the body's tissues and transported through the blood to a target tissue, where it acts to produce a specific response.

neurotransmitter – A chemical substance that provides a signal to receptors located throughout the body.

glycogen – The form of glucose that is stored in the muscle and liver.

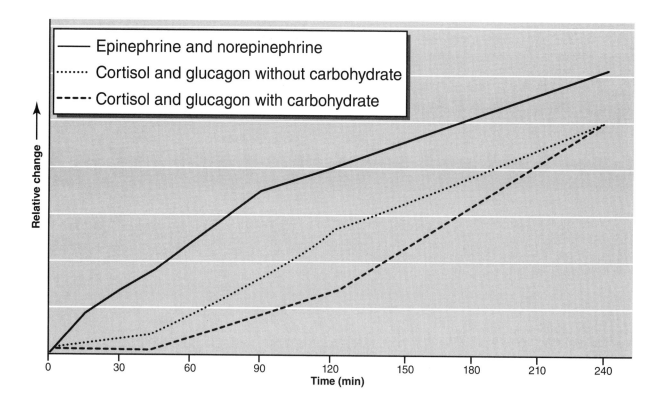

Figure 1.1 Responses of epinephrine, norepinephrine, cortisol, and glucagon to exercise. Note that cortisol and glucagon levels increase during exercise. In the absence of carbohydrate, the increase in these hormones is sharp, but with carbohydrate ingestion, the increases in the levels of cortisol and glucagon are slower and more moderate.

the body's tissues. During exercise, insulin allows glucose to be readily used by the body's working tissues. The sensitivity of the muscle cells to insulin increases when exercise is stopped.

The actions of cortisol and glucagon are dependent on the amount of glucose in the blood and on energy availability in the body. Glucagon is increased in response to low blood glucose levels; it is responsible for breaking down carbohydrate stored as glycogen in the liver and facilitating the conversion of amino acids to glucose. Cortisol is the hormone that facilitates the synthesis of glucose from the breakdown of protein and fat in times of a reduced energy state. When blood glucose levels drop too low during exercise, glucagon is increased to promote glycogen release from the liver and, if necessary, works with cortisol to promote the synthesis of glucose from free fatty acids and amino acids.

Muscle Regeneration

A number of factors—from enzymes, to blood flow, to receptors on the muscle cell, to hormone action—are elevated to the greatest extent in the first 45 minutes after exercise stops. Over the next several hours, these factors slowly return to resting levels; thus, the 45 minutes after exercise is considered a window of opportunity for the ingestion of foods that will promote muscle recovery through glycogen replenishment and rehydration.

This response is highly facilitated by the enzyme glycogen synthase and a transporter known as **GLUT4**, both of which are responsive to insulin and are significantly elevated after exercise. Together glycogen synthase and GLUT4 enhance the uptake of carbohydrate and improve glycogen storage. These actions are further facilitated through insulin, which facilitates carbohydrate uptake and increases the rate of muscle blood flow. This not only helps deliver nutrients to the muscles but also aids in the elimination of metabolic waste that was produced during exercise. In the 45 minutes immediately after exercise, the activity of GLUT4 receptors and levels of glycogen synthase are maximally elevated, allowing insulin to facilitate carbohydrate restoration to the muscle cells and improve recovery from training (figure 1.2).

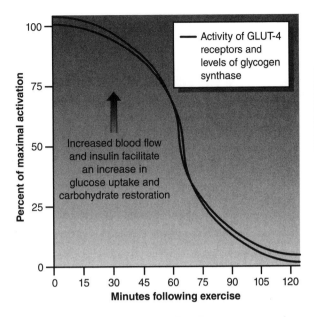

Figure 1.2 The activity of GLUT4 receptors and levels of the enzyme glycogen synthase are significantly elevated in the first 45 minutes after exercise, then begin to decline rapidly.

GLUT4 – A receptor that is located in skeletal muscle, the heart, and fat and is highly regulated by insulin. It is responsible for the uptake of glucose.

Types of Carbohydrate and Protein

The functionality of foods is covered in greater detail in chapter 4, but it is important to note here that intake of the right type of carbohydrate is significant evidence for timing nutrient ingestion. In addition, the timing of protein and the type available to the muscle are critical for optimizing adaptations from resistance and cardiovascular training.

As mentioned, insulin is an important hormone in the muscle response after exercise. The rate of posttraining muscle glycogen synthesis has been shown to be proportional to the increase in blood insulin levels. Athletes should therefore select the type of carbohydrate they consume based on how quickly glycogen stores must be replenished, which depends on the amount of time between training sessions. When the next training session will begin determines the type of carbohydrate and insulin response that is desired. For most athletes, muscle glycogen can be sufficiently restored through the use of low to moderate glycemic carbohydrates that do not require a significant spike in insulin and will steadily restore glycogen. This approach will also help to minimize gains in body weight. An example of a postexercise snack that would provide this response is whole wheat bread with almond butter and banana. When glycogen restoration must happen quickly, the best types of carbohydrate to stimulate an increase in blood insulin levels are those that evoke a high **glycemic response** because of their rapid conversion to glucose in the blood. An example of a postexercise snack that would provide this response is white bread with banana and honey. All are made of simple sugars and have minimal fiber content so that digestion and absorption by the body can be done quickly. The more readily glucose can become available to the working muscles, the faster the rate of glycogen resynthesis can occur and recovery can begin. This is frequently the case for athletes who perform

glycemic response – A measure of a food's ability to raise blood glucose.

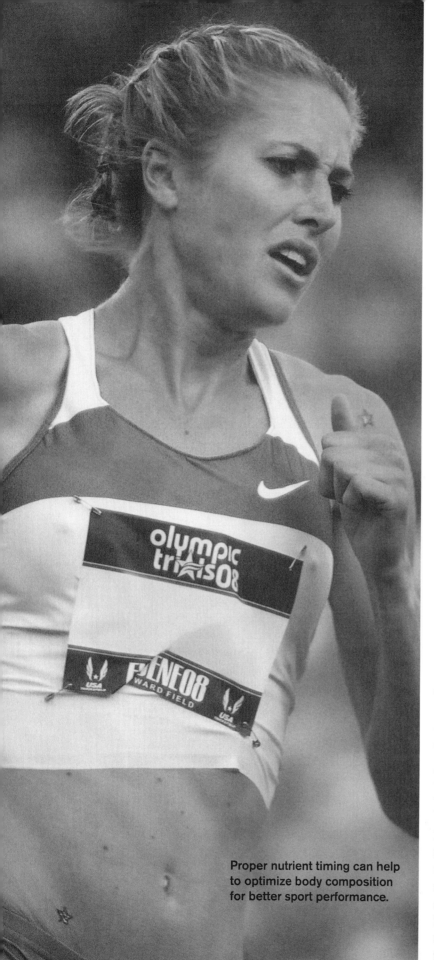

Proper nutrient timing can help to optimize body composition for better sport performance.

multiple prolonged training bouts within a day or, in the case of a weight-classified sport, athletes who must replenish glycogen stores from having cut weight.

Glycogen restoration may be further enhanced through the ingestion of protein with carbohydrate. This is attributed to the optimization of the insulin response and the suppression of cortisol, which speeds the muscle's recovery process. The availability of essential amino acids (such as those found in dairy and meat products) before and after training is also an important factor in maintaining or increasing muscle protein synthesis. Thus, it is important that the protein source used contain all the essential amino acids. Depending on an athlete's food preferences, this can be accomplished by consistently consuming foods in the daily diet that contain all the essential amino acids or by ensuring that the pre- and posttraining snack contains foods that are a good source of essential amino acids.

Body Composition

Most athletes seek to optimize the ratio of muscle and fat mass in the body because of the positive relationship this has with performance. Studies assessing the patterns of food intake by athletes have shown that eating meals at regular intervals is most optimal for maintaining a high level of muscle mass and a lower level of body fat. These same studies show that most athletes eat infrequently and consume a majority of their calories in a large meal at the end of the day. This leads to large rises in blood glucose that in turn encourage the storage of fat mass. Furthermore, this eating pattern delays energy restoration, and so the body utilizes muscle proteins to make and maintain blood glucose levels, leading to a decrease in muscle mass. For the body to optimize its composition, blood glucose needs to stay stable. When an athlete consumes the energy expended in a training session through frequent eating that revolves around training, the muscles are functionally available and ready to absorb the nutrients ingested, thus helping to maintain stable levels of glucose in the body. Timing nutrient ingestion revolves around the supply and demand for energy production by the working body, which enhance body composition. Improvements in body composition result in an improved ratio of muscle mass to fat mass and in turn directly result in an improved work capacity.

Nutrient Timing, Training, and Performance

Now that we have established the basis for timing nutrient ingestion, it is important to understand the physiological principles that support its use. This means understanding how the body regulates food intake, what limits performance, the goal of training, and how to use the principles of recovery and adaptation as the foundation for improving sport performance.

Using Nutrient Timing to Optimize Training Adaptations

Human work capacity is considered to be limited primarily by the muscles' capacity to do work. Improvements in performance come as a result of progressive overload, which can be imposed through increases in the volume, frequency, intensity, or perception of work. The body is stressed by a training load (and other life stressors such as work, school, friendships, and relationships), and the work undertaken results in a degree of fatigue or depletion of the physical or psychological systems involved. Performance gains are accelerated when fatigue is reduced as soon as possible after training and the challenged systems are restored to normal levels. Learning to accommodate a training stressor (i.e., load) can eventually lead to successful adaptation. An athlete's nutrition must be seen as a tool in this process. By understanding the principles of recovery and adaptation, and how food or the lack thereof can be a performance-limiting factor in these processes, you can begin to understand the positive role food can play in the training program.

Recovery and Adaptation

The primary goal of recovery is to overcome muscle fatigue and establish a greater ability to generate power. The principle of recovery can be defined as the part of training where the benefits of the work done are maximized through practices that reduce fatigue and enable the athlete to cope with the training load more effectively. Recovery is about encouraging adaptive processes after the presentation of a training load. If there is sufficient recovery before the next workload, the underlying system or fuel store stressed during training can improve its capacity to cope with the next stressor. To maximize an athlete's potential to learn, adapt, and improve, it is important to start training and competition in a relatively nonfatigued state. This becomes more challenging for coaches and athletes when athletes are required to complete more than one training session per day, often over several days, and when combined with a range of additional lifestyle stressors such as education, work, and so on.

Adaptation can be defined as the body's response to a stressor that has thrown the body out of homeostasis (i.e., balance). The body's response to a stressor can be positive or negative adaptation, and this adaptation can be short term (minutes to hours) or long term (days to weeks). A positive adaptation will result in an improved function by the body (e.g., increased sweat rate during exercise in the heat), and a negative adaptation is seen as a plateau or reduced capacity of the body (e.g., reduced sweat rate after heat stress). It is thought that the cumulative effects of multiple short-term adaptations will result in a long-term adaptation.

By thinking of food in the context of creating short- and long-term training adaptations, you can begin to understand the interrelation of training and nutrition with performance. Food is a key part of sufficient recovery before the next training session; food restores the energy system that was stressed during training so it can improve its capacity to cope with the next stressor. Ensuring restoration of fuel stores facilitates adaptation to an imposed stressor. When this is done appropriately, an athlete can begin the next training session in a state of energy regeneration, and an additional stressor can then be imposed. The overall effect is to improve training and cause faster adaptation (figure 1.3).

Monitoring Training

Assessing the progression of an athlete's adaptation to an imposed training stressor is important because it provides a measurable outcome that indicates whether or not the body is adapting favorably to training. A training stressor or nutrition intervention is valuable only if the outcome is an improvement in work capacity or some other measure of performance. These assessments can be objective (physiological tests designed to evaluate the effects of an intervention) or subjective (feedback from the athlete). Ideally they are used in combination to measure the progression of adaptation to training. Most frequently, recovery and adaptation are assessed through blood markers that measure energy use; cardiovascular capacity; and immune, hormone, and enzyme function along with the athlete's feeling of perceived exertion and total body recovery (psychological, physiological, and muscular).

How might this relate to timing nutrient ingestion? Often an athlete can perceive the benefits of a nutrition program only when it is compared with training under less than ideal nutrition practices; thus, monitoring training allows an athlete to evaluate the benefits of an intervention. The examples of hydration and recovery nutrition are probably the simplest and best ones we have found to date. In the case of hydration,

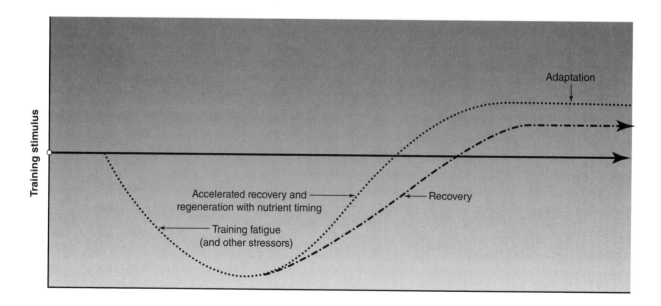

Figure 1.3 With proper nutrient timing, accelerated recovery from each training session leads to more effective adaptation to the stress of training.

an objective measure of heart rate over the training bout provides evidence that heart rate and thus cardiovascular strain is less in a hydrated state when compared with training in a state of dehydration. To examine the effects of postexercise nutrition, an athlete should train for several days without eating and drinking immediately afterward and then evaluate muscle recovery and readiness for the next training session. When the athlete repeats this experiment with the ingestion of postexercise carbohydrate and protein (food or drink), there will be a definite pattern of improved readiness to complete the next training bout. Monitoring training is beneficial because it allows the athlete, coach, and support team to evaluate the effectiveness of a nutrition intervention or of training load stressors.

Framework for Timing Nutrient Ingestion

From the previous sections, it can be seen that timing nutrient ingestion is about using food to support the physical training process. As a result, the framework for timing nutrient ingestion revolves around three key time points: before, during, and after training. The timing of intake and the type and volume of food necessary to support training are dependent on the volume and intensity of the last training session completed and the period of time an athlete has between sessions. This is the first step for each athlete: determining the daily training schedule and what steps to take to ensure that food intake can support the training sessions. In determining the composition and volume of food intake at each of these time points, an athlete must ask several questions. How quickly do I need the fuel? How is the fuel going to be utilized? What is the purpose of the training cycle and session? How much time is there before the next training session? The concepts in this section will be covered further in chapter 6, which discusses ingestion of the different macronutrients before, during, and after training, and in chapter 4, which looks at the functionality of foods.

Timeline

The timeline for nutrient ingestion before training can further be divided into greater than 2 hours, less than 2 hours, or less than 1 hour before training. The timeline for after training can also be further divided into less than 45 minutes, less than 2 hours, and greater than 2 hours after training. When considering nutrient ingestion during training, it is very important that the goal of the training session be identified and then further refined based on intensity and duration. During training bouts of high-intensity exercise, where the goal is to optimize the body's ability to utilize carbohydrate, consumption of carbohydrate is appropriate; conversely, when the goal of the training session is to improve the body's ability to utilize fat as a fuel source, then refraining from carbohydrate intake may be appropriate for some athletes during certain times of the training year.

Type of Food

When thinking about the type of food needed before, during, or after training, the most important thing you must remember if you are an athlete is that only you know what works best for you! Everyone has a different response to food because we all have unique digestive systems. This book provides the guidelines, but it is up to the athletes to take them to the next level and customize them to their bodies with specific details.

The foods chosen at various time points are heavily centered on the body's response to a rise in blood glucose, which is termed the *glycemic response*. The glycemic response is a measure of the rate at which a food or meal will cause a rise in blood glucose. A high-response food or meal results in the rapid conversion of a food into glucose, and a low response results in a slow and prolonged time period for converting food into glucose. Thus an athlete must ask, "How quickly do I need the fuel?" This may bring to mind the terms *glycemic index* and *glycemic load*. Both of these terms are covered in greater detail in chapter 4, but for now, the term *glycemic response* is best used to address the type of food needed along the training timeline.

Preexercise Fueling

Choosing a preexercise snack or meal can be challenging depending on an athlete's schedule and the availability of food choices. It is important, however, to maintain a steady rate of glucose coming into the bloodstream of the body. Preexercise food choices should be aimed at avoiding the "spike and crash" pattern of blood glucose change known as rebound hypoglycemia.

The best type of meal or snack to eat before training is one that will digest easily. Carbohydrate and protein should be the predominant sources of energy, with low levels of fiber and fat. Fluid ingestion should be evenly spread out before, during, and after a meal to aid in digestion and promote hydration to carry an athlete through the workout and into the recovery period. Fluid intake must be based on sweat rate and individually calculated.

Absorption of the meal is often dependent on how long an athlete has before training. When there is more than 2 hours before training, a meal with a moderate to low glycemic response is recommended. This in turn also helps optimize the insulin response to glucose. Meals and snacks that are moderate to low in their glycemic response will minimize any sharp rises in insulin since they cause a slow and steady release of glucose into the blood. Though a meal with moderate to low glycemic response is a good general guideline, research examining the effects of different glycemic meals in this time frame has shown very little difference in performance for meals ranging from a low to high glycemic response. Therefore, athletes should choose meals based on what works best for them. Athletes who are prone to gastrointestinal discomfort should consume a meal that is moderate to high in glycemic response before training to speed digestion, or be sure that the low glycemic carbohydrate consumed is of a high molecular weight (i.e., waxy maize or superstarch) and can easily move out of the stomach. See chapter 6 for more on the use of these specialized carbohydrate sources.

As the timeline comes closer to training and there is less than 2 hours, consuming food that helps to maintain a steady blood glucose response is desired. Less than an hour before training, it is best to consume carbohydrate snacks that are rapidly absorbed. The volume of carbohydrate consumed at this time point is important in the insulin response. These foods usually have a high glycemic response, and if too much is consumed, they will cause a large increase in insulin. Just before training, it is important to ensure that insulin does not spike, as this may cause a performance disadvantage by increasing the rate of carbohydrate usage too early in training, leading to early muscle fatigue; however, this can be eliminated by ingesting carbohydrate during exercise.

Fueling During Exercise

During exercise the goal is to sustain energy so that training quality can remain high. This means ensuring that carbohydrate consumed during exercise can move through the stomach and into the bloodstream without causing any form of distress to the athlete. The types of foods best suited for ingestion during exercise are those with a high glycemic response or foods that can produce a low glycemic response as a result of a high molecular weight carbohydrate and not cause GI distress. Carbohydrate is usually used alone during exercise, unless it is exercise of prolonged endurance in which case the ingestion of amino acids may be beneficial. In sports where mental concentration and maintaining a lower heart rate are desired, it may also be important that protein or some form of amino acids be available to help prevent psychological fatigue and to help control blood glucose levels.

Carbohydrate should be consumed during training only when the duration is greater than 60 minutes and is of high intensity or when the focus is the sustainability of a high-quality work output. In today's world, this message has been overridden by the advertisement of carbohydrate supplements boasting performance gains from their consumption during exercise. However, it is important to remember training goals and that most of the studies examining carbohydrate and performance used a one-trial scenario. In other words, researchers did one performance trial without carbohydrate and another trial with carbohydrate, and *then* it enhanced performance. The subjects were not chronically adapted! If the body becomes accustomed to carbohydrate consumption during exercise, that long-term adaptation can offset any gains in performance on competition day. When fuel intake is sufficient before and after training, athletes do not need to be concerned with glycogen depletion depending on the duration and intensity. It is more important to ensure proper hydration to maintain blood volume and reduce the cardiovascular strain on the body.

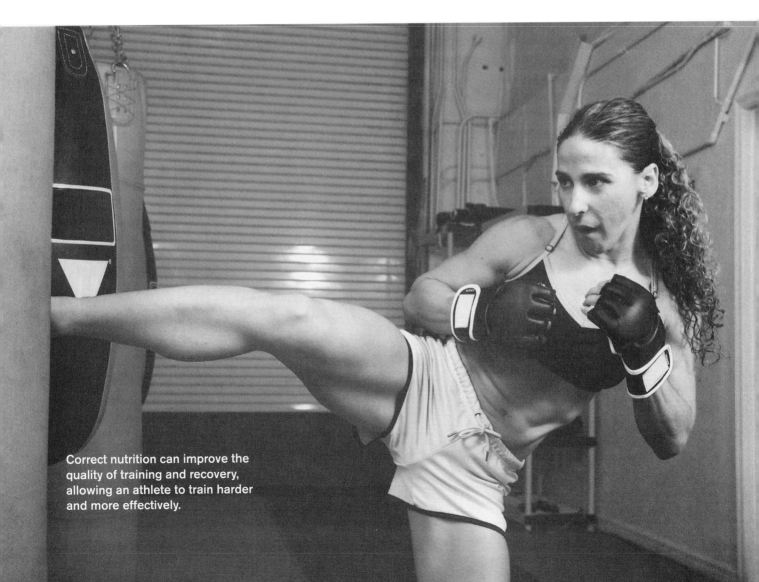

Correct nutrition can improve the quality of training and recovery, allowing an athlete to train harder and more effectively.

Postexercise Fueling

To optimize training adaptations, it is important that an athlete restore the fuel that was depleted during a training session. Foods to be consumed after exercise need to be easily transportable and must not require refrigeration. Restoring energy to the body at this time is frequently best accomplished through foods that are not subjective to the environment (heat or cold) and can easily be opened and consumed without any need for a cooking device. In the 45 minutes after exercise, carbohydrate foods and drinks and protein have been shown to quickly restore muscle glycogen. After this 45-minute window and over the next 2 hours, athletes should continue consuming snacks or meals that have a low to moderate glycemic response rate. The choice of foods is dependent on when the next training bout is scheduled. For the remainder of the day (unless another training bout is scheduled within 4 hours), the consumption of mixed meals and snacks that elicit a moderate to low glycemic response is appropriate; most of these meals or snacks easily maintain stable blood glucose levels.

Nutrient Timing, Food Intake, and Body Composition

Body weight and composition are a result of the balance between food intake and energy expenditure. More important for an athlete is the concept of energy flux, which is the rate at which energy is consumed in relation to the rate at which it is expended, whether through daily living or exercise. Athletes desire a high energy flux, which has been shown to help improve body composition through increasing muscle mass gains and decreasing body fat. To achieve this, an athlete must develop a timing system that increases the rate of energy intake and expenditure. Examples of days with high and low energy flux are shown in figure 1.4.

Hunger and Satiety

hypothalamus – Found in the upper portion of the brain stem, the hypothalamus is responsible for the control of many physiological processes, including food intake (hunger and satiety).

For years practitioners have used quantitative methods such as counting calories to assess energy balance, but the body in and of itself does not sense or measure energy flux by this means. Rather, it is the input of the **hypothalamus** in the central nervous system that determines energy stores—and signals when food is necessary to maintain body weight—and other processes such as muscle repair and rehydration. In the same sense, the hypothalamus can also drive what type of macronutrients the body desires to eat and when. This is something we refer to as instinctive eating. Instinctive eating is when we learn to listen to our bodies in terms of when, what, and how much to eat and drink. This is covered in greater detail in chapter 3, where the psychology of eating is discussed.

In the brain, there are two centers that control the sensations of satiety and hunger. Satiety is the desire and satisfaction component of food intake, and hunger is the sensation of appetite and fullness (i.e., when an adequate amount of food has been ingested). Neurotransmitters appear to control these areas and thus determine food intake. Feedback from the gastrointestinal (GI) tract can also indicate hunger, and expansion of the GI tract results in suppression of the hunger center in the brain. The blood also influences hunger signals. A drop in blood glucose will signal hunger, whereas a rise in free fatty acids in the blood will signal fullness. Together, these signals provide the means for using instinctive eating to determine the frequency of food intake (figure 1.5 on p. 12).

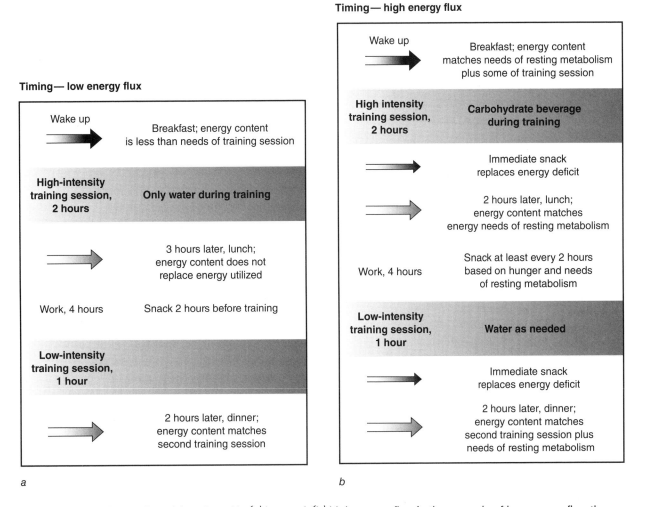

Figure 1.4 A sample training day with *(a)* low and *(b)* high energy flux. In the example of low energy flux, the energy content of food is inadequate to meet the demands of training. In the example of high energy flux, energy intake matches training needs.

Instinctive eating results in athletes eating frequently throughout the day. This not only helps maintain stable blood sugar and insulin levels but also results in a greater energy flux and thus a higher metabolic rate. Together, this translates into athletes being able to eat more and store less fat. When athletes do not eat frequently and allow the body to go into a state of starvation, metabolic rate is decreased to compensate for the lack of energy supply, and fat is stored. If this continually occurs over time, the body will lower its metabolic rate in preparation for periods of energy deficit, and even when the athlete is eating normally the body will store more fat. Thus, eating before hunger sets in is important. Blood sugar is known to rise and fall in 3-hour periods, so the concept of timing nutrient ingestion relies on time frames of 2 to 4 hours to ensure that blood sugar does not maintain a sustained drop at any point throughout the day.

Volume of Food

Traditionally, athletes have been encouraged to examine the volume of their food intake based on calories and a percentage of carbohydrate, protein, and fat intake.

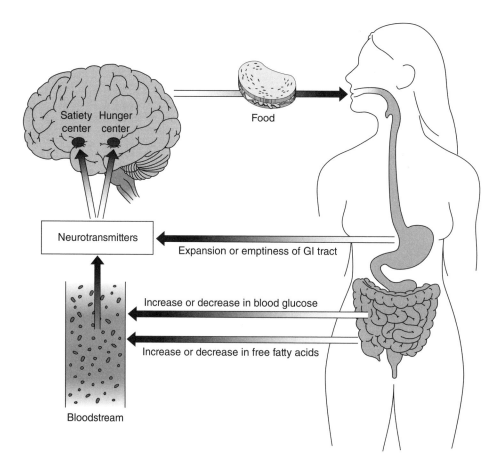

Figure 1.5 The brain relies on feedback from neurotransmitters, the GI tract, and blood glucose to signal hunger and fullness.

Other methods also include examining carbohydrate and protein intake based on grams per kilogram (g/kg) of body weight and duration of training each day; however, athletes are rarely willing to calculate these numbers on a day-to-day basis, and many would need to be in dire straits before they would do so. Although the value of caloric or macronutrient analysis cannot be discounted, the goal is to provide multiple options because not all athletes operate in the same fashion. In addition, most recommendations based on body weight apply only to athletes that are approximately 110 to 176 pounds (50 to 80 kg). Although this covers a wide range of athletes, many athletes fall well outside this range. As a result, a basic integrated quantitative and qualitative approach to timing nutrient ingestion is presented here. In later chapters, further information regarding carbohydrate, protein, and fat is given based on type of sport.

The qualitative aspect of timing nutrient ingestion is mainly focused on those time points that occur outside of training. The application of this concept is highly dependent on the ability to tap into instinctive eating, which is further discussed in chapter 3. Athletes can achieve a healthy mix of foods by paying attention to how much of the plate is covered by different types of food. For both meals and between-meal snacks, one-half of the plate should be fruits and vegetables, one-quarter of the plate a protein source, and one-quarter of the plate a carbohydrate in the form of a whole grain or starch.

The quantitative component of timing nutrient ingestion falls before, during, and immediately after exercise. Recommendations are dependent on the type of training being performed (cardiovascular versus resistance training) and, for competition days, on the demands and logistics of the sporting event. The timing of carbohydrate and protein intake affects both training adaptations and immediate performance.

The quantitative approach to nutrient timing calls for both meals and snacks to be calculated based on caloric needs as determined through estimates of energy expenditure or based on recommended ranges of carbohydrate and protein intake that have been derived based on volume of training. Determining energy expenditure is a function of caloric needs at rest and during exercise, the processing of a meal, and activities of daily living. Figure 1.6 summarizes the factors used to build an athlete's nutrition timing plan. Total caloric intake can be spread throughout the day into several small meals and snacks that are centered around training. In the same sense, this can be done using grams to calculate carbohydrate and protein intake over the day. Table 1.1 provides the most current recommended ranges for carbohydrate and protein intake based on volume of training per day. Chapter 2 goes into further detail on energy assessment and how to determine caloric needs.

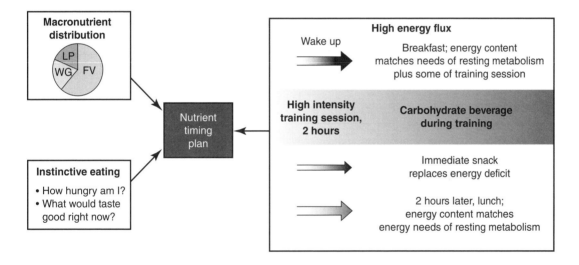

Figure 1.6 Energy flux, timing of nutrient intake, instinctive eating, and the need to distribute macronutrients (by balancing intakes of lean protein, whole grains, and fruits and vegetables) to meet an athlete's goals all come together in a nutrient timing plan.

Table 1.1 **Recommended Ranges of Carbohydrate and Protein**

Training duration	Carbohydrate (g/kg/day)	Protein (g/kg/day)
Up to 1 hour/day	4-5	.8
1-2 hours/day	5-7	1-1.2
2-4 hours/day	7-10	1.2-1.4
4-6 hours/day	10-12	1.2-1.7

Conclusion

As you can hopefully see, the concept of timing nutrient ingestion is not just about the food an athlete eats; it is also necessary to understand the body's response to a training demand. Through synchronizing training with nutrient intake, an athlete and coach can see how all these factors work together to improve performance. If you are an athlete, what are your training goals? If you are a coach, what are the training goals of your athlete? Identify the top three, and see if a performance nutrition plan that supports these goals can be formulated by the time you have completed this book.

Assessing Sport Performance

To design the most effective nutrition program, you must identify the goals and objectives of the training cycle. This is best done by first performing a needs analysis of the sport or athlete. Coaches and athletes frequently use information from books, magazines, and other sources of media to guide their nutrition programs, often without determining what type of athlete the information is applicable to. Understanding an athlete's needs and evaluating whether something is appropriate are the keys to ensuring an effective nutrition program. When assessing an athlete's sport, you must determine how performance can be improved in order to know how nutrition can be implemented to make a difference. To truly make a difference in performance, you need to assess and evaluate the effects of training on the body through physical testing and performance analysis. In addition, you must bring together all other aspects of training and find the appropriate balance that allows for full integration of the nutrition plan into the bigger picture.

The needs analysis should include an evaluation of the sport's physical demands and culture and the athlete's own unique background and needs. The following list of questions can be used by a fitness professional or coach to guide the aspects of a needs analysis and summarize what is observed:

- What energy systems are most used in the athlete's sport?
- What factors are critical to the athlete's performance success?
- How will changes in nutrition affect the athlete psychologically?
- Based on the age of the athlete, what type of nutrition intervention is appropriate?
- To achieve the nutrition goals, what type of behavior change may be necessary?
- How much time will be needed to achieve the athlete's nutrition goals?
- Are there any financial limitations to achieving the nutrition goals?
- What type of springboards can be used to help move the athlete forward, and what type of obstacles might get in the way?

- If there are obstacles, what solutions might be readily available to move the athlete forward? Are there springboards that can be used to overcome these obstacles?

- How much education will be necessary to help the athlete achieve the goals?

- Should an educational approach be taken with the athlete rather than one that is prescriptive?

- Who surrounds the athlete, including parents, support staff, and friends, that may need to be educated so that a sound environment is provided to support the nutrition plan that is to be implemented?

- What is the interaction between coach and athlete in regard to nutrition? Is it positive or negative?

- Is there performance testing in place, and does it track the effects of training and the nutrition interventions?

- Does the assessment need to include tests for body composition, force production, reaction time, agility, strength, and aerobic or anaerobic capacity? Does any type of psychological assessment need to be performed?

- What is the athlete's competition schedule? How does the athlete need to prepare for each competition site?

- What type of environment needs to be created to achieve optimal success with the athlete's performance and nutrition goals?

Sport Performance Analysis

The first step in a needs analysis is to understand the physical demands of the sport and how this influences an athlete's performance. This can be done through analysis of specific skills that indicate performance quality (i.e., that distinguish higher and lower levels of athlete performance) and, for nutrition purposes, through identification of the energy systems and how they are used.

A needs analysis also involves an understanding of how other areas of sport science come into play. Examples include (1) whether the athlete needs to carry extra body weight to obtain a strength or cardiovascular training adaptation (e.g., a wrestler or endurance athlete), (2) whether a higher level of body fat (and thus potentially weight) is more advantageous in maintaining body position in training and competition (e.g., an endurance swimmer or heavyweight rower), (3) whether training without carbohydrate is needed to improve fat utilization (e.g., endurance athlete or sprint swimmer), and (4) whether an athlete can handle the recommended fluid intake during training or competition because of sport-specific movement (e.g., boxing or another combative sport). Optimizing the concept of timing nutrient ingestion involves taking these types of aspects into consideration. The whole basis for timing nutrient ingestion is recovery and adaptation to training; thus, training goals often dictate what the nutrition goals will be. These issues also demonstrate the need for periodization of the nutrition plan, which is covered more specifically in chapter 7.

Determining the Energy System

To determine a sport's predominant energy system, several questions must be asked. How long does the event last? Is the event performed continuously? If not, what is the balance between the ratio of work and rest? What is the intensity of the work being performed in training and competition?

Three primary energy systems are used to classify the physical demands of a sport. Energy is supplied in the form of **ATP (adenosine triphosphate)**, and the source of ATP is dependent on the rate at which it must be supplied to the working muscles. Adenosine triphosphate can be produced without oxygen, known as anaerobic metabolism, or with oxygen, known as aerobic metabolism.

Anaerobic metabolism is a function of the **ATP–CP (creatine phosphate) energy system** and anaerobic glycolysis. The ATP–CP system is limited to the phosphates found in the muscle cell itself and thus only predominates in sport events that are approximately 10 seconds long, such as the long jump or 100-meter sprint, or that require repeated bouts of up to 10-second bursts (i.e., anaerobic endurance), such as basketball, soccer, wrestling, taekwondo, tennis, and most other team and combative sports (figure 2.1). Athletes training for explosive **power** rely on this energy system.

Anaerobic glycolysis is the second energy system the body can immediately recruit to supply energy during high-intensity events. The energy supply comes from glycogen that is stored in the muscle cell and glucose that is readily available in the blood. This energy system predominates during events that last from 10 seconds up to 3 minutes, such as the 800 meters (track), 400 meters (track and swimming), rowing, kayaking, canoeing, and downhill skiing (figure 2.1). A by-product of anaerobic glycolysis is lactic acid, which ultimately becomes the rate-limiting factor in the performance of this energy system. As lactic acid accumulates in the muscle and blood at high concentrations, the muscles' ability to contract and produce force becomes limited. Hydrogen ions generated from lactic acid inhibit muscle crossbridge formation and thus force

ATP (adenosine triphosphate) – Energy; universal currency of the human body.

ATP–CP energy system – The energy system that uses creatine phosphate (CP) stored in the muscle; used to supply ATP in the absence of oxygen for short, intense bursts of exercise.

power – Force multiplied by velocity; the rate at which work is done.

anaerobic glycolysis – Energy system that works via conversion of glucose to ATP in the absence of oxygen. Lactic acid is a by-product of this system.

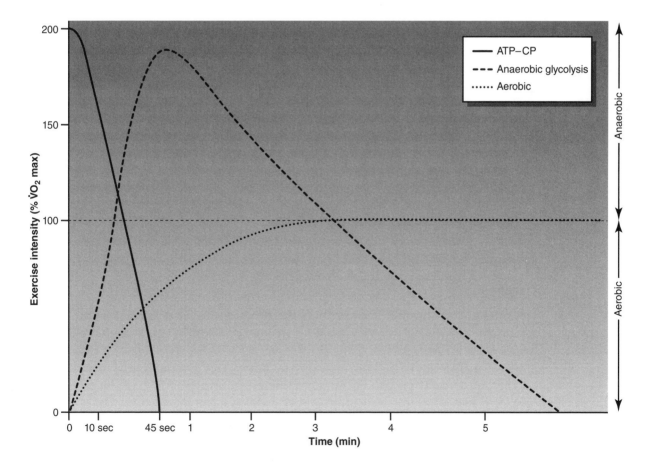

Figure 2.1 All three energy systems provide energy, but their relative importance changes depending on the duration and intensity of the activity.

aerobic energy system – System that works in the presence of oxygen to produce ATP from fat and carbohydrate stores.

mitochondria – The powerhouse of the muscle cell that is responsible for making much of the body's ATP.

production. Athletes looking to maximize this energy system train for strength and power and must learn to tolerate high levels of lactic acid. This is done by developing the muscle's buffering capacity to tolerate lactate.

The **aerobic energy system** is the energy pathway that produces ATP from glucose, glycogen, fat, and protein during exercise intensities that can be sustained for greater than 3 minutes. It is the most efficient of the energy systems because of the high yield of ATP produced by the powerhouse of the muscle cell, the **mitochondria.** Mitochondria can generate the largest amount of ATP from glucose and fat stores because of the high levels of oxidative enzymes that are contained within its pathways, which generate energy very efficiently. Aerobic metabolism predominates in endurance events requiring a continuous supply of oxygen (figure 2.1). The greater the number of mitochondria that arise from training, the better an athlete can generate ATP from fat and improve the capacity of this energy system. Aerobic metabolism is rarely limited by the availability of fuel during exercise; rather, it is limited by the athlete's ability to sustain force. Therefore, endurance athletes continuously try to reduce the amount of lactic acid produced and improve their resistance to muscle fatigue.

Performance is limited not by the energy systems themselves but by the capacity of the skeletal muscle to repeat a movement over and over again. There are two primary types of muscle fibers: Type I and Type II. Type I fibers are known as slow-twitch muscle fibers; they have high capabilities for aerobic energy production because of their ability to use oxygen. Characteristics of this type of muscle fiber include low resistance to fatigue and a slower rate of contraction and force production than Type II fibers. With aerobic endurance training, this muscle fiber type can increase the levels of carbohydrate and fat stored, increase the density of mitochondria and enzymes responsible for the use of these fuel sources during exercise, and improve oxygen delivery through increases in capillary density and as a result increase the ability of the muscle to utilize oxygen. Athletes who participate in endurance events are characterized by higher percentages of Type I fibers.

Athletes who participate in events that are more highly dependent on anaerobic energy sources demonstrate a higher percentage of Type II fibers. These fast-twitch muscle fibers have a high contraction velocity but fatigue quickly. Type II fibers have two subgroups: Type IIa and Type IIb. Both of the subgroups have a high capacity to store carbohydrate and the potential to support the anaerobic energy systems. However, Type IIa, while highly fast twitch, also has the means to support aerobic metabolism. With different types of training, the ability of Type II fibers to adapt to a more aerobic (IIa) or anaerobic (IIb) capacity has been shown.

The type of training and the shift in skeletal muscle function that an athlete is looking to achieve are important in the interpretation of nutrition for the enhancement of performance. Nutrition should be designed to enhance the characteristics of the different types of muscle fibers so that training and nutrition intake is optimized. This is why it is critical to understand what energy system the athlete is working on developing in each day of training.

Often two athletes with similar capabilities will get to their performance using totally different means—that is, they utilize different ratios of the energy systems to achieve the same end result. This underlies the importance of understanding the energy system that is creating the performance (figure 2.2) and tailoring nutrition programs to fit each person. For example, in an 800-meter track event, one athlete may use the aerobic energy system for 70 percent of the effort, and another may use the anaerobic system for 70 percent of the effort, yet both can run the same time. Frequently, this is based on what type of workouts the athletes are good at accomplishing. The more aerobic

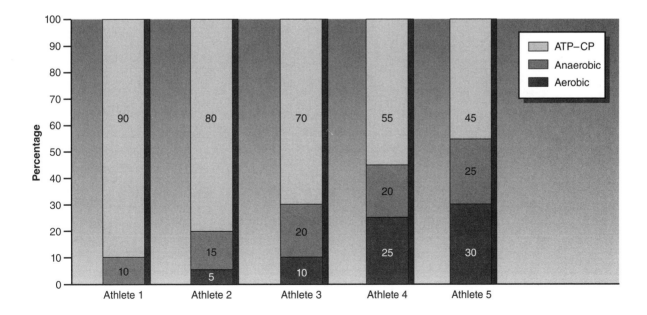

Figure 2.2 Athletes can obtain similar performances through a variation in use of the energy systems. The key is to understand the contribution of each energy system and provide nutrition support that is appropriate for the training volume and intensity necessary for optimal performance.

athlete can perform repeated 400-meter strength and endurance work with shorter recovery times, whereas the anaerobic athlete requires more rest but can run a faster 100 and 200 meters than the athlete who is more aerobic. The energy systems work on a continuum to supply the fuel necessary for performance, and depending on the duration of an event, there is always one that will predominate. Table 2.1 gives a list of the energy systems and the activity duration and source of energy production associated with each.

Athletes as Individuals

A key part of a needs analysis is determining who athletes are as individuals. Usually athletes can be defined by far more than just the sport they play. Do they have a unique ethnic background? What foods do they enjoy? Do they have to balance kids, work, and family life? What are their priorities in life? More important, what defines them is a key part of how they get to their own performance. As a result, it is important that athletes be empowered to "drive" their nutrition program. Empowered athletes can rationalize what their goals should be and determine their own timelines for nutrient ingestion, along with using instinctive eating to guide their food choices.

The people working with an athlete to promote or identify nutrition change must be aware of how willing or ready the athlete is to do so. The behavioral change required for nutrition is multifactorial and complex; it may involve multiple changes in training, food choices, and responses to stimuli, and it affects many aspects of a person's daily life.

Health and Nutrition Status

Before an athlete implements any changes in nutrition habits or goes through performance testing, it is import to perform a review of overall health. The physical evaluation of who an athlete is as an individual should consider at least the following issues: biological and chronological age, sex, current training, training background, age in the sport, and nutrition history. It should also include any acute or chronic illnesses, musculoskeletal injuries, or other medical issues (allergies, cardiovascular and pulmonary health). This assessment must be thorough enough to minimize any physical risks to the athlete.

From a nutrition standpoint, a nutrition history such as the one provided in figure 2.3 (pp. 22-23) should be completed. The history should include the reason for nutrition changes; a record of body weight and composition; any nutrition strategies, food patterns, timing, and food intake in relation to training schedule and type of training performed; supplement use; menstrual cycle regularity; and any performance test recently completed. It may also include an assessment of cooking skills and any

Table 2.1 **Energy Systems for Activities Based on Duration**

Duration	Classification	Predominant energy supply
1 sec to 10 sec	ATP–CP	ATP (in muscles) + creatine phosphate
10 sec to 2 min	Anaerobic	ATP (in muscles) + creatine phosphate + muscle glycogen
2 min to 4 min	Anaerobic + aerobic	Muscle glycogen + creatine phosphate + lactic acid
4 min to 5.5 min	Aerobic + anaerobic	Muscle glycogen + fatty acids
>5.5 min	Aerobic + anaerobic	Fatty acids + muscle glycogen

Examples of Determining the Energy System

ATHLETE 1

Sport Details

Sport: Ice hockey

Physical demands of sport: Short bursts of speed on the ice for up to 2 minutes should the athlete complete a full shift. This is repeated throughout the game.

Duration: An athlete's time spent on the ice is dependent on the ability to score, defend, and recover from the previous bout.

Energy Systems

Primary energy system: ATP–CP system

Secondary energy system: Anaerobic glycolysis during competitive plays on the ice. The aerobic energy system is utilized during recovery.

Muscle fibers to target: Training to increase the capacity of Type II muscle fibers is critical for success in the sport.

ATHLETE 2

Sport Details

Sport: Ice dancing

Physical demands of sport: Balance, coordination, core stability, speed, and high anaerobic capacity

Duration: 4 to 6 minutes on average

Energy Systems

Primary energy system: ATP–CP system

Secondary energy system: Aerobic system. Some bursts of activity will be long enough in duration to call upon the anaerobic glycolysis system.

Muscle fibers to target: Training to increase the capacity of Type II and Type I fibers must be done to accomplish the energy capacity the athlete will need.

---

other issues of food preparation that may need to be addressed before the start of a program. Depending on the type of information needed, a nutritionist may also obtain estimates of caloric intake and quantity and quality of the macronutrients as they relate to the athlete's daily schedule.

Vegetarian Athletes

The term *vegetarianism* is used loosely by many athletes, from those who just do not eat red meat to those who do not eat any animal products at all. Some of the more common categories of vegetarian diets include the following:

- Lacto-vegetarian: No animal foods at all but includes milk and milk products (yogurt, cheese, cottage cheese).
- Lacto-ovo-vegetarian: No animal foods at all but includes eggs, milk, and milk products.
- Vegan: No animal foods at all.

Nutrition History

Name:_____ Age:_____ Gender:_____ Date:_____

Body height:_____ Body weight:_____ Sum 7 or Body fat %:_____

Contact information: _____

_____

Medical History

Current medical concerns: _____

_____

Medications and supplements: _____

_____

History: Please list any medical issues you have had regarding your heart, blood, lungs, bones, joints, and muscles.

Heart (blood pressure, chest pains, fainting, murmurs, and so on): _____

_____

Lungs (difficulty breathing, asthma, allergies, and so on): _____

_____

Blood (iron stores, glucose, diabetes, electrolytes): _____

_____

Bone, muscle, or joints: _____

_____

Menstrual history: _____

_____

Current Nutrition Practices and Goals

Primary nutrition goal: _____

Key strategies for performance: _____

_____

From K. Austin and B. Seebohar, 2011, *Performance nutrition: Applying the science of nutrient timing* (Champaign, IL: Human Kinetics).

Training	Monday	Tuesday	Wednesday	Thursday	Friday	Saturday	Sunday

D = Duration; I = Intensity

Morning							
	D:	D:	D:	D:	D:	D:	D:
	I:	I:	I:	I:	I:	I:	I:

Afternoon							
	D:	D:	D:	D:	D:	D:	D:
	I:	I:	I:	I:	I:	I:	I:

Favorite Foods

Breakfast	Lunch	Dinner	Snacks
1	1	1	1
2	2	2	2
3	3	3	3
4	4	4	4
5	5	5	5

Please answer the following questions:

Do you enjoy cooking? _____

How well do you know how to cook? _____

Do you prepare your food in advance? _____

Anything you would like to share:

_____

_____

_____

_____

_____

Figure 2.3 A form like this may be used to gather information about an athlete's health, training schedule, and food preferences.

From K. Austin and B. Seebohar, 2011, *Performance nutrition: Applying the science of nutrient timing* (Champaign, IL: Human Kinetics).

Athletes who follow any form of vegetarian diet seem to have a lower risk of developing diseases such as diabetes and heart disease when they get older, and although there isn't much support for improved performance, since vegetarian diets are usually high in carbohydrate, performance is typically improved. However, a few areas of interest should be noted by athletes embarking on or already practicing some form of vegetarianism.

Most vegetarian diets are high in carbohydrate-rich foods such as fruits, vegetables, and grains, which are packed with fiber. This can contribute to a higher sense of feeling full, which can result in not consuming enough calories to support training and competition. If this happens, an easy strategy to fit more calories into an athlete's eating program is to include more calorie-dense foods such as nuts and nut butters.

Protein intake could be low if vegetarian athletes do not eat animal meat or dairy foods and are not familiar with other foods that contain good sources of protein. Good options for vegetable protein include nuts, tofu, soy products, rice and almond milk, whole grains, cereals, and beans.

Iron stores are of utmost importance for any athlete, specifically females who practice vegetarianism and who have regular menstrual cycles. Iron is needed to transport oxygen to muscles, and lower stores could have a negative effect on performance and recovery from training and environmental stresses such as altitude. Nonanimal sources of iron include spinach, broccoli, almonds, oatmeal, and iron-fortified cereals. This is discussed in more detail in chapter 9.

Other micronutrients, specifically calcium and vitamin B_{12}, are also of concern. For those vegetarian athletes who do not drink milk or consume dairy foods, calcium stores may be low, which can affect bone health and muscle stimulation. Alternate sources of calcium-rich foods include fortified cereals and milk, tofu, and green leafy vegetables. There is no active form of vitamin B_{12} in plant foods, and because this vitamin is involved in the breakdown of foods to energy, insufficient amounts can be detrimental to performance. Vegan athletes are at risk of developing anemia from deficiency of this vitamin, which can lead to fatigue. Fortified foods are the top choice and include cereals and soy products.

It is possible to follow any type of vegetarian eating program and still be healthy and perform well. The important message is that vegetarian athletes must add more variety and choose many options of fruits, vegetables, nuts, legumes, soy products, and meat alternatives.

Pregnancy and Nutrient Timing

Many active females continue their training programs during the first and second trimesters of pregnancy with great success. During the third trimester, females usually have to stop their training and focus on physical activity that will not promote ill feelings or exercises that are safe for the expectant mother and baby. Some nutrition changes are required during the three trimesters of pregnancy. The traditional daily increase of 300 to 500 calories holds true in some females, but the extra caloric load is highly individual and should be customized to the pregnancy progression and exercise needs. Lactation also requires an additional caloric intake, around 500 calories per day, but should also be customized based on individual preferences and situations.

Related to nutrient timing and nutrition periodization, maintaining blood sugar should top the list to ensure the fetus receives the nutrients it needs for proper growth. A small carbohydrate and lean protein snack should be included 1 to 2 hours before each exercise session to stabilize blood sugar. Additionally, fluid needs are increased slightly, and it is important to remain hydrated throughout the day and enter exercise sessions fully hydrated so that dehydration is minimal. Consuming 3 to 8 ounces (90 to 240 ml) of fluid every 15 to 20 minutes during exercise is recommended.

Psychological and Social Aspects of Eating

It is also important to evaluate the psychological viewpoint that athletes have toward food and who they are as persons. Rarely is food choice as physically based as it appears; what drives an athlete's eating style is what must be understood. Altering food intake is a very personal and intimate thing. Thus, before anyone can successfully commit to a nutrition plan, that person needs to accept that change is necessary, and the environment must be right to support that change. The psychological aspects of nutrition are discussed in depth in chapter 3. It is important for a needs assessment to include an evaluation of the athlete's personal attitudes and social environment.

A sport's culture often plays a significant role in how athletes interact with food. Frequently the culture associates food with training, performance, and social interaction. Some athletes are accustomed to consuming alcohol on a nightly basis, whereas others would see this as taboo unless outside of the training season. In some sports, the level of an athlete's body fat is not readily paid attention to, whereas in others it is viewed as such a disadvantage to performance that an increase in body fat or weight results in instant criticism or rejection by other athletes. Within each sport's culture, there is a key person who typically is leading or influencing what is done. For most athletes, this is the coach, followed by teammates, family, and friends. Younger athletes are usually most influenced by their parents. Nutrition is dependent on how these people view its role in performance and how they will work to support the changes required.

The ability to succeed in sport is dependent on having the support to do so; thus, environment is a key component to success. In terms of food, the environment encompasses everything from culture to time, friends, family, support staff, and finances. So what influences an athlete's food intake? What is the athlete's history with food? What kind of food is accessible? What kind of time constraints need to be considered? Are there financial limitations that will influence what is eaten? What is needed for success? What positives are present that could assist and negatives that would deter? Figure 2.4 shows some of the diverse factors that affect an athlete's food intake.

Identifying what or who influences the athlete's take on food is the first step in reaching the tipping point toward change. The environment an

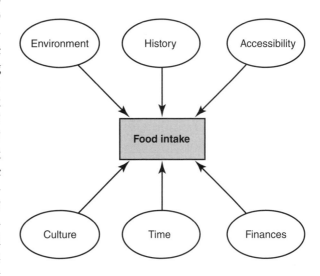

Figure 2.4 Many factors contribute to what an athlete will eat on a daily basis. Making food choices is rarely dependent on any one factor but rather is a result of multiple influences.

athlete functions in needs to support and promote what is best for that athlete. This includes those who will hold the athlete accountable and help ensure success. Each person is different, and the process of creating the optimal environment must be individualized. The support team's role is to educate and provide the athlete with the tools necessary to achieve the goals. This may initially involve helping the athlete be empowered and have the confidence to tell the team what the athlete needs. Often the role of a supporting team member is being a voice of reason or just knowing when to help the motivated athlete hold back from doing too much. If an athlete is not empowered, creating a sense of empowerment is the first step for success!

Creating a Toolbox for Performance Nutrition Assessment

The toolbox for assessing performance nutrition is often created by a collaborative group of people (a performance-enhancement team) who serve as the support team around the athlete. The performance-enhancement team will work with tools associated with macronutrient and micronutrient status and the energy systems. The tools provided here are divided into those associated with **work capacity** and energy systems, monitoring the training load, energy intake and expenditure, body composition and somatotype (body type), blood markers, and fluid balance.

work capacity – Ability of the body to produce work of different intensity and duration using the energy systems of the body.

Work Capacity and Energy Systems

Performance testing monitors changes in the physical work capacity of an athlete due to training or a given intervention. The more specific the testing is to the sport and the greater it characterizes changes in training, the more effectively it can evaluate the energy systems an athlete is using. Performance nutrition strategies should result in an improved work capacity, and at times they may be the only intervention taken to do so. Examples include alterations in the timing of when an athlete consumes a pre- or postexercise snack to improve body composition and work capacity as well as changes in the type of macronutrients consumed and when they are consumed so as to promote the use of fat instead of carbohydrate during submaximal exercise intensities. In some instances, testing may be used to evaluate weight loss or gain or changes in dietary composition and their impact on training or key measures of performance.

It is important to appropriately match testing for work capacity to a sport's energy system. Performance analysis can help identify the key characteristics associated with improved work capacity. Tests can then be selected that match the key physical demands of the sport, and these same tests can be used to monitor progress in response to a nutrition intervention. Performance analysis and testing can be done through descriptive means such as time–motion analysis, comparison between energy systems used in competition and training, heart rate monitoring, and global positioning systems (GPSs). Time–motion analysis provides descriptive information such as distance covered at various speeds during a match, the number of unforced or forced errors an athlete may have made, the number of seconds between high-intensity efforts, the number of foot strikes over a set distance, the use of various techniques to score on an opponent, and how an athlete paced a race. Heart rate monitoring can be used to evaluate the time spent at a given percentage of maximal heart rate as well as to evaluate work-to-rest ratios or the ability to recover. Global positioning systems can examine factors such as maximal speed or percentage of maximal speed, rate of acceleration or deceleration, distance covered, and average speed. Together, these tools can be used to choose appropriate testing and to monitor progress. The sidebar on page 28 describes an example of how various analysis and testing tools might be used in a nutrition intervention for a field hockey player.

Testing can also assess training and its focus, and whether changes need to be made to accommodate a strength or weakness in the athlete's work capacity. The Performance Tests sidebar on page 29 lists tests for evaluation of performance by energy system.

Anaerobic Power and Capacity

Performance tests for anaerobic power and anaerobic capacity examine metabolism involved in short-duration, high-intensity performance. Power is the maximal rate at which work can be done. Anaerobic power is considered to be reflective of the ATP–CP energy system. It is measured by peak power and is usually related to kilograms of body weight. Anaerobic capacity is considered to be a measure of anaerobic glycolysis and is evaluated by average power, average power produced per kilogram of body weight, a fatigue index, maximal heart rate, and the amount of lactate an athlete can produce and tolerate while performing at high intensity.

A good example would be the characteristics required to successfully perform in the sport of wrestling. Athletes must be able to complete one-off power movements to overcome their opponents as well as repeatedly take their opponents down and hold them with great strength. To improve in this sport, athletes must increase maximal power (one-off explosive movement), increase average sustainable power (to repeatedly overcome the opponent), and minimize fatigue (as indicated by percentage of decline in power from maximum to average and minimum over a given time period). This requires tolerating high levels of lactate and performing at a high percentage of maximal heart rate throughout the match while also recovering as quickly as possible. Recovery can be indicated by how well the athlete is removing lactic acid and by how quickly heart rate returns to resting levels.

Aerobic Power

Measures to examine aerobic metabolism and working capacity include maximal oxygen uptake ($\dot{V}O_2$max), anaerobic threshold, exercise economy (oxygen use and carbon dioxide production), respiratory exchange ratio (RER), and heart rate. These tests are traditionally performed on athletes involved in endurance events. $\dot{V}O_2$max is the maximal amount of oxygen that can be used by the working muscles. Anaerobic threshold is the highest exercise intensity that can be performed without a predominance of the anaerobic energy system. Exercise economy is the fraction of oxygen relative to maximum that is needed to perform a submaximal workload. The RER during exercise is reflective of the relative percentage of fat and carbohydrate used at a set workload. Heart rate has a direct relationship to measures of oxygen consumption and is assessed because of its practical use in the field for quantifying energy expenditure and training load.

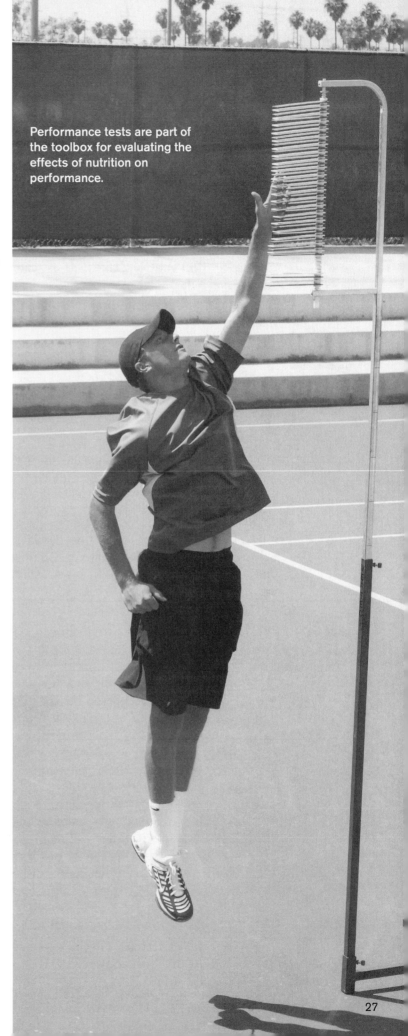

Performance tests are part of the toolbox for evaluating the effects of nutrition on performance.

Performance Analysis and Testing

Athlete: This athlete consistently becomes fatigued during competition, and it has been suggested that carbohydrate intake may need to be increased to ensure sufficient energy supply. The athlete currently takes in approximately 15 grams of carbohydrate in each 35-minute period through a carbohydrate and electrolyte beverage. Fatigue does not occur in training sessions.

Sport: Field hockey. This sport is characterized by intense bursts across a field and is played in two halves of 35 minutes each.

Time–motion analysis: Use to measure the amount of time spent jogging, standing, and sprinting during a game as well as how many sprints are performed consecutively.

Comparison of competition to training: Use to measure the amount of time spent utilizing each energy system as well as the work-to-rest ratio that occurs in training versus competition.

Heart rate monitoring: Use to measure the cardiovascular demands of competition, including amount of time spent at a relative percentage of maximal heart rate and the time it takes for heart rate to recover after intense bouts.

Global positioning system: Use to measure the distance an athlete covers in competition. In addition, it can help determine training volumes for conditioning purposes.

The best tests for determining the carbohydrate needs of an athlete and the impact an increase in carbohydrate supplementation would have are time–motion analysis and the comparison between energy systems used in competition and training. Two factors must be considered to understand why an athlete is fatiguing during competition. The first is how much carbohydrate needs to be consumed and how frequently during the game; the second is whether or not the fatigue may be a result of improper conditioning for the demands of competition. To understand the performance improvement from carbohydrate, intake during the next competition could be moved up to 1 gram per minute (i.e., 35 grams per half), and testing could be repeated to determine the effects of the nutrition intervention.

Endurance training should result in an increased oxygen use by the working muscles and therefore an improved ability to make ATP through the mitochondria of Type I muscles. Thus any intervention (training or food intake) that results in an improvement of the muscle's endurance and the use of fat as a fuel source should result in an improved economy, as reflected by a lower amount of oxygen used at a set workload and a reduced reliance on carbohydrate. An example is the aerobic power necessary to perform successfully in an event such as a marathon. Athletes must learn to produce more power with each foot strike while also conserving glycogen stores. This can best be accomplished by teaching the athlete's body to utilize fat as a fuel source. The amount of fat and carbohydrate that is contributing to an exercise bout is traditionally determined by a treadmill test, where RER is measured as part of the aerobic power assessment. If the training or nutrition intervention has been successful, an athlete will require less carbohydrate to perform the same submaximal workload, and instead fat will be utilized as the fuel source. This can also be seen by the fact that an athlete will not need as many revolutions per minute (frequency of foot strike) to cover the same distance at a given speed.

Anaerobic Endurance

In sports such as volleyball, badminton, soccer, and wrestling, energy is derived from more than just one energy system and is more highly dependent on the ability of the

Commonly Used Performance Tests

AEROBIC ENDURANCE

Lactate profile + max test (power, speed, or stroke rate)

Submaximal oxygen uptake (power, speed, or stroke rate)

$\dot{V}O_2$max

1- to 3-mile (1.6 to 4.8 km) run

6-minute run

2,000-meter row

1,000-meter swim

Wheelchair aerobic test

Kosmin test

AGILITY

Illinois Agility Run

Zigzag test

Agility cone drill

Quadrant jump test

505 agility test

Shuttle run

20-yard (18.3 m) agility test

Hexagon test

T-test

STRENGTH

1RM, 2RM, and 3RM tests

Abdominal strength tests

Straight-leg abdominal strength test

Isokinetic strength tests

Burpee test

Wall squat

Push-ups

Pull-ups

Sit-ups (30 seconds versus 2 minutes)

POWER

Vertical jump

Standing long jump

Three-hop test

Margaria-Kalamen test

10-second versus 30-second Wingate test

40-meter cycle sprint

30-meter acceleration

SPEED

Flying 30-meter test

20- to 60-meter sprint (swim or run)

Sprint from A to B (duration of <10 seconds)

300-meter run

400-meter drop-off test

10-stride test

150- to 250-meter speed endurance test

ANAEROBIC ENDURANCE

Running-based anaerobic sprint test

3 × 300-meter anaerobic running economy

Wingate test (6 × 10- to 30-second repeats)

800-meter run

500-meter row

450-meter swim

Cunningham and Faulkner treadmill test

athlete to repeatedly explode and recover from intense bouts that require such characteristics as speed, agility, strength, stamina, and power. In these sports it is important to understand what percentage of maximal intensity can be sustained repeatedly with short recovery periods. It is necessary to be able to tolerate high levels of lactic acid and remove it in a timely manner while also being able to sustain a high level of work output. Research has shown that fatigue during intermittent exercise is not related to a lack of energy or the accumulation of lactate; rather, it is thought that muscle fatigue occurs because the motor units responsible for telling the muscle to contract become fatigued, decreasing drive from the brain to the muscle.

Increases in strength and muscular endurance are related to improvements in sustainability within the aforementioned sports. As maximal strength is improved, each submaximal level of work should become progressively easier to maintain. Thus performance testing should be directed toward evaluating maximal strength and power, functional strength (the ability to sustain a given amount of work over and over again), the rate at which functional strength can be sustained, and lactate tolerance and clearance. An example is the sport of ice hockey. Athletes must repeatedly sprint at high velocities throughout the game. To accomplish this, an athlete must be able to repeatedly contract the muscles at a very high level of power output. A test for repeated sprint capability over a given distance will indicate whether training or nutrition intervention is improving the athlete's ability to sustain power output and functional strength. This is applicable because the test is sport specific, and it also requires an improvement in work capacity in order to achieve a better score.

Monitoring the Training Load

Work capacity is assessed to monitor changes in an athlete's physical capacity in response to an intervention. To understand whether the addition of carbohydrate or another intervention was beneficial, work capacity must be assessed before and after the intervention, and the training load the athlete was able to tolerate while implementing the nutrition strategy must be determined. To optimize the information gained from these assessments, it is important to monitor the training load imposed and the athlete's response to this load. A training load is traditionally calculated to assess the effects of training, but it can also be used to understand the effects of a nutritional intervention. A method for doing this is known as a TRIMP (training impulse). A TRIMP is based on the volume and intensity of training. It is calculated for each training session, day, and week by multiplying the duration of training by the rate of perceived exertion (RPE) (table 2.2) for that session. To further account for the athlete's psychological view on the training session, a satisfaction score can be incorporated; this is shown in the training and recovery monitoring sheet. An example can be seen in table 2.3. A depiction of the calculated training load for each session is found in figure 2.5 and each day's total in figure 2.6. Information that can and

Table 2.2 **RPE Scale**

RPE number	Breathing rate/ability to talk	Exertion
1	Resting	Very slight
2	Talking is easy	Slight
3	Talking is easy	Moderate
4	You can talk but with more effort	Somewhat hard
5	You can talk but with more effort	Hard
6	Breathing is challenged/don't want to talk	Hard
7	Breathing is challenged/don't want to talk	Very hard
8	Panting hard/conversation is difficult	Very hard
9	Panting hard/conversation is difficult	Very, very hard
10	Cannot sustain this intensity for too long	Maximal

Table 2.3 Example of Tracking a Training Impulse (TRIMP)

Date	Training duration 1	RPE 1	Satis-faction 1	TRIMP score 1	Training duration 2	RPE 1	Satis-faction 1	TRIMP score 2	Total TRIMP
1	30	2	3	60	5	10	1	50	110
2	15	8	4	120	20	8	5	160	280
3	8	10	1	80	35	3	6	105	185
4	60	2	7	120	15	10	2	150	270
5	20	5	9	100	7	5	9	35	135
6	13	7	10	91	60	1	10	60	151
7	5	9	3	45	20	3	3	60	105
Average	21.6	6.1	5.3	88.0	23.1	5.7	5.1	88.6	176.6

Duration = minutes and does not include recovery time.

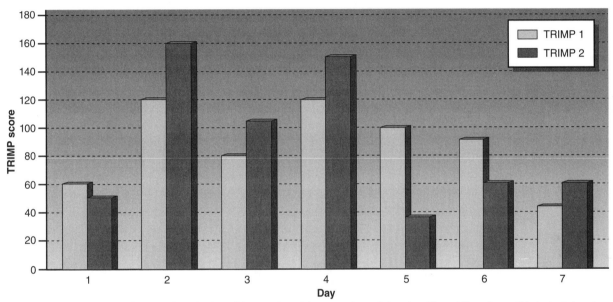

Figure 2.5 A TRIMP score is calculated for each training session of the day. The ability of an athlete to tolerate a training load can best be determined by comparing this to the recovery score obtained on the following day.

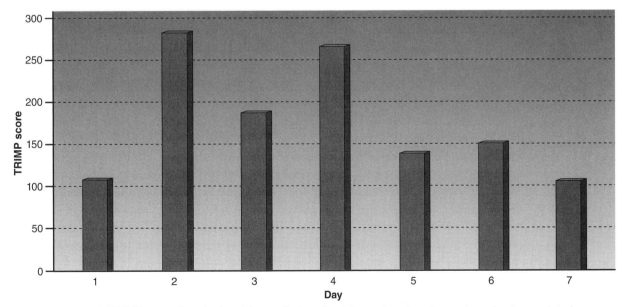

Figure 2.6 A TRIMP score is calculated for each day of training rather than for each workout completed. Understanding the athlete's training load can be achieved through either method.

should be derived from the training load includes the criterion for a training effect, the minimum load that will produce a desired training effect, and the maximum possible training load. It is often necessary to monitor several training cycles so these criteria can be determined. Objective tools such as heart rate, distance covered, and time should also be tracked, along with additional subjective measures of training and overall well-being.

The goal of monitoring training is to ensure that training sessions induce an increase in the need for energy from the energy system of focus and that acute and long-term adaptation occur so that the body can function at a higher level of work capacity. In addition, monitoring training ensures that once adaptation has taken place, further training does not lead to overtraining. Although it is appropriate that athletes intentionally overreach (a transient incompetence in performance) for a short period of time, overtraining results in a loss of the training adaptation and a regression in performance that cannot be overcome without substantial time off from training.

Factors such as heart rate and time are excellent objective measures of adaptation to training, but the impact of training or the training load is also dependent on the athlete's perception and awareness of how the session is going. Thus, it is also appropriate to include subjective measures of training. With so much technology in today's world, coaches often forget to simply ask the athlete how a training session felt. When training and everything else in life are going well, the athlete can perceive training appropriately or even easier than it is intended to be. Conversely, when training or other aspects of life such as social influences, school, weather, or illness are not optimal, perception of a training session can be much harder than the actual muscular and cardiovascular demand. As a result, subjective measures that can include a comparison rating; resting heart rate; total recovery score; individual scores for physical, muscular, and psychological recovery; quality of sleep; hours of sleep; and mood state should be taken into account when evaluating training and work capacity. A training and recovery tracking sheet is shown in figure 2.7.

Assessing Energy Intake and Expenditure

The components of energy expenditure that are of the most value are the resting metabolic rate (RMR) and respiratory exchange ratio (RER). Resting metabolic rate is a measure of the caloric needs at rest. Caloric needs at rest are dependent on several factors including age, body size, body composition, training status, menstrual cycle (for female athletes), and most important, genetics. The RER is a measure of the type of fuel burned while at rest; it ranges from .7 to 1.0 and is highly dependent on training and the composition of an athlete's food intake. The value of .7 is reflective of the body's sole reliance on fat metabolism, and the value of 1.0 indicates that the body is utilizing carbohydrate for fuel. Values in between are reflective of relying on a combination of fat and carbohydrate. For example, a value of .85 shows a mixed utilization of carbohydrate and fat. Depending on the goal of the nutrition program, an athlete may attempt to improve the use of carbohydrate or fat in training or at rest. Timing nutrient ingestion can be a means to shift metabolism toward carbohydrate or fat utilization by manipulating the type of fuel available around training.

Both RMR and RER are measured via a method known as indirect calorimetry. For this assessment, an athlete most likely will need to find a performance testing laboratory that is linked to a university or high-performance training center. Testing involves the use of a metabolic hood that measures the oxygen consumed and the carbon dioxide produced by the body. The volume of oxygen consumed per kilogram

Training and Recovery Monitoring Form

Athlete: _____   Resting heart rate: _____

No. hours slept: _____   Quality of sleep: _____

Muscle recovery: _____   Mental recovery: _____   Total quality: _____

Satisfaction scale _____   Training duration: _____ (hh:mm:ss)

Rate of perceived exertion: _____   Comparison rating: _____

Recovery Scale

0	No recovery
1	Extremely bad recovery
2	Very bad recovery
3	
4	Bad recovery
5	Recovery OK
6	Good recovery
7	
8	Very good recovery
9	Extremely good recovery
10	Maximal recovery

Rate of perceived exertion

1	Very slight
2	Slight
3	Moderate
4	Somewhat hard
5	Hard
6	Hard
7	Very hard
8	Very hard
9	Very, very hard
10	Maximal

Comparison Rating*

1	No difference
2	
3	Some difference
4	
5	Different
6	
7	Noticeably different

Satisfaction scale

0	Best workout ever
1	Very satisfied
2	
3	Fairly satisfied
4	
5	Neither
6	
7	Fairly dissatisfied
8	
9	Very dissatisfied
10	Worst workout imaginable

*Comparison is made to the same or a similar workout, and a difference is dependent on the improved ease the athlete has in completing the training session.

Figure 2.7   This form can be used to monitor training load and recovery using subjective measures.

From K. Austin and B. Seebohar, 2011, *Performance nutrition: Applying the science of nutrient timing* (Champaign, IL: Human Kinetics).

of body weight is used to determine caloric needs. The ratio of oxygen consumed to carbon dioxide produced determines the RER.

The RMR can also be estimated through regression equations that take into account a person's height and weight. Some equations also include age. The equation that is most relevant to the athletic population is one developed by Delorenzo and colleagues:

$$-857 + 9 \text{ (weight in kg)} + 11.7 \text{ (height in cm)}$$

Using RMR and RER for the purpose of timing nutrient ingestion is solely to evaluate the effects of training and shifts in energy use. Differences in training intensity and energy system focus can affect these measures, and nutrition should equally match these changes. Resting metabolic rate provides a baseline of caloric intake that an athlete must meet daily. Although this does not account for training and activities of daily living, the proper use of hunger and satiety should allow an athlete to increase and decrease caloric intake appropriately. Most important, RER provides an indication about shifts in fuel use. Thus, as the RER moves closer to .7, the diet should include more fat; conversely, it should include more carbohydrate as the RER moves closer to 1.0. When teaching the body to rely on a different energy source at rest, the composition of what is eaten needs to assist in this shift.

In some instances, athletes may choose to use estimates of energy expenditure in relation to energy intake to further control dietary intake. Total energy expended can be estimated through the addition of RMR, an activity factor (AF), and energy expended during training. An AF accounts for the activities of daily living and can be estimated by multiplying RMR by the AF as listed in table 2.4.

Energy expenditure in training is dependent on the sport and whether it is more aerobic or anaerobic in nature. Energy expended through aerobic metabolism can be determined by assessing oxygen uptake through indirect calorimetry while the athlete is performing the particular mode of exercise. This typically requires testing in a laboratory setting. For every liter of oxygen utilized per minute during exercise, it can be assumed that approximately 5 calories are burned. The relationship between heart rate and oxygen uptake allows for daily estimates of the athlete's energy expenditure through a heart rate monitor. This method assumes a predominant use of the aerobic energy system and thus is most appropriate for activities that are performed continuously for at least 3 minutes.

Events in which strength and power predominate rely heavily on anaerobic metabolism in which energy is produced without oxygen. Many of these activities are dynamic in nature and cannot be performed in the laboratory setting. In the research literature there is a compendium of physical activity that provides caloric expenditure in the form of metabolic equivalents (METs). The MET value can then be multiplied by the athlete's body weight and duration of time spent training to estimate the calories expended. The article by Ainsworth and colleagues listed in the bibliography section for this chapter compiles a list of METs.

Table 2.4 **Activity Factor**

Activity level	Activity factor
Sedentary (little or no exercise, desk job)	1.2
Lightly active (light exercise/sports 1-3 days/week)	1.375
Moderately active (moderate exercise/sports 3-5 days/week)	1.55
Very active (hard exercise/sports 6-7 days/week)	1.725
Extremely active (hard daily exercise/sports and physical job or training twice a day)	1.9

It is also important to consider subjective measures when evaluating energy intake. Assessing how well the size and composition of a meal creates fullness and satisfaction is important when looking to optimize the response a person feels toward food. The hunger and satiety scales provided in chapter 3 (p. 45) can be used to evaluate a known amount of calories and meal composition, and the desire to eat along with the potential for further food consumption can also be assessed. When satiety is high and hunger low after a meal, the size and composition of the meal were right for the person; this can greatly aid in designing the food content of meals. The response can vary depending on increases or decreases in energy expenditure, and realizing this helps an athlete control food intake when changing the volume of training.

Assessing Body Composition and Somatotype

Body composition can be used to evaluate an athlete's performance as it relates to the amount of work produced or oxygen utilized per kilogram of fat-free mass, which can in turn help determine whether increasing or decreasing fat-free mass would benefit the athlete. Evaluating body composition is also important for health purposes, but it cannot directly predict performance—a wide range of body compositions has been associated with successful performance within the same sport. However, for most people, there is a ratio of muscle mass to fat mass that is associated with their best performance. Research has found an inverse relationship between fat mass and activities requiring the ability to carry body weight over a distance that is vertical or horizontal. Athletes must learn to evaluate their body composition based on their own personal ranges, which should be tracked over an entire training and competitive season. The goal is to identify the body composition that allows for optimal performance without injury or a loss of health. Nutrition to optimize body composition is best when food is consumed around training. An athlete can optimize performance by providing energy to the body at the appropriate time points in the training schedule.

Dual-energy X-ray absorptiometry (DEXA) is considered the most accurate and appropriate way to evaluate body composition (figure 2.8). It assesses regional (arms, legs, and trunk) and total fat and fat-free content of the body's tissues as well as regional and

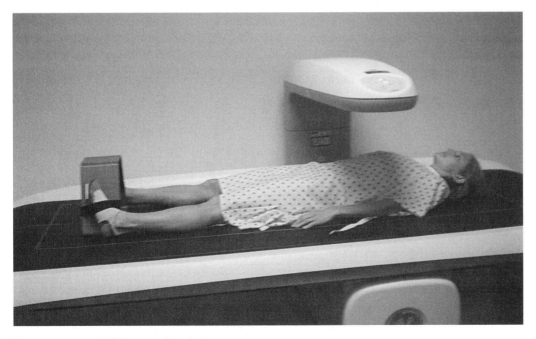

Figure 2.8 DEXA scanning device.

Photo courtesy of Krista Austin.

total bone mineral content. Athletes can track regional and total changes in grams of fat mass as it relates to total body weight in grams. This method of assessing body composition requires travel to a university or hospital laboratory and has a higher cost (US$150 to $200).

Several less expensive and portable methods are available to assess body composition; the most valuable method that can be easily used in the field is anthropometry. Anthropometry is the measure of skinfold thickness and circumference. Skinfold thickness is an estimate of subcutaneous (external) fat mass and is measured using calipers that report thickness in millimeters (figure 2.9). In conjunction with circumference measurements, skinfolds can determine whether there have been changes in muscle mass and fat mass. A reduction in skinfold thickness where the circumference of a muscle has stayed the same or increased indicates an improvement of muscle mass.

The International Society for the Advancement of Kinanthropometry (ISAK) publishes the most recognized standard for anthropometry techniques. Its technique examines eight different skinfold sites (triceps, subscapular, biceps, iliac crest, supraspinal, abdominal, front thigh, and medial calf) and six circumferences (arm [relaxed], arm [flexed and tensed], waist [minimum], gluteal [hips], calf [maximum], and thigh) in the standard profile. The information obtained can be used to monitor body composition by two different methodologies. The sum of skinfold sites indicates relative amounts of body fat in comparison to normative data that have been gathered on various sports. The individual skinfold values provide information on sites of fat storage, and the changes in values on subsequent measurements show the effects of training or a nutrition intervention. The differences can be examined as an absolute or relative percent change.

A second use of skinfolds incorporates mathematical equations to predict a percent body fat. The equations are highly dependent on the group (age, sex, ethnicity, training status) for whom they were derived; thus, it is important to ensure that the equation used is appropriate for the athlete. Since these equations can only estimate body fat and can potentially be significantly skewed, it is recommended that percent body fat not be provided to athletes unless it is necessary. This is best demonstrated by choosing two different mathematical equations that are intended for the same population and comparing the percent body fat obtained. The difference in scores generated by the two separate equations will show why percent body fat should be avoided if possible. Although use of this methodology should be minimized, there are times (e.g., estimating weight reduction) when it is appropriate.

Somatotyping examines body shape and composition. It can be used to understand the long-term development of an athlete's body and how changes in nutrition intake may help shape an athlete's physique. Somatotyping includes not only the assessment of skinfolds and girths but also genetically determined measures such as bone breadths and limb lengths. It is often used to compare various levels of athletes, characterize physique changes over an athlete's life span, or compare the relative shapes of athletes in different sporting events. A somatotype gives a quantitative summary of an athlete's physique. It is expressed as a three-number rating representing endomorphy, meso-

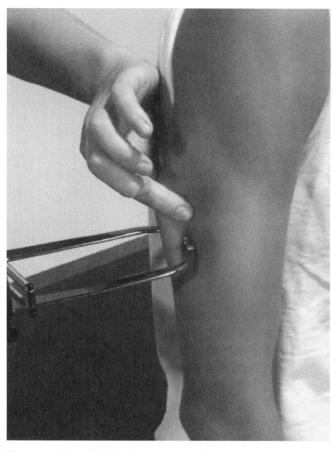

Figure 2.9 Skinfold measurement.
Photo courtesy of Jean Lopez.

morphy, and ectomorphy—endomorphy indicating fatness, mesomorphy indicating muscularity, and ectomorphy indicating linearity or slenderness. When a body shape can be associated with a sport, it is usually considered to be a result of natural selection.

The Heath-Carter somatotype method is internationally recognized and has been used to collect and quantify data on athletes. The abbreviated method of assessment requires measurement of stature, body mass, four skinfolds (triceps, subscapular, supraspinal, medial calf), two bone breadths (biepicondylar humerus and femur), and two limb girths (arm flexed and tensed, calf). Endomorphy, mesomorphy, and ectomorphy are then calculated and plotted on a somatograph (figure 2.10).

Blood Chemistry for Health and Performance

In monitoring training, blood markers can be a valuable tool when paired with information on phase of training, training load, and subjective markers of overall well-being and recovery. Ideally, blood profiles are taken with every change in the training cycle. Markers can then be divided into two categories: those associated with health and those associated with performance. Blood markers can be examined by two means, the first of which is to compare them to standard medical reference ranges. The second is to examine values relative to the athlete's own range. A combination of these methods is preferred because it takes into account individual variability and response as well as reference ranges for good health. The most common markers are listed in table 2.5 along with their possible use in monitoring training.

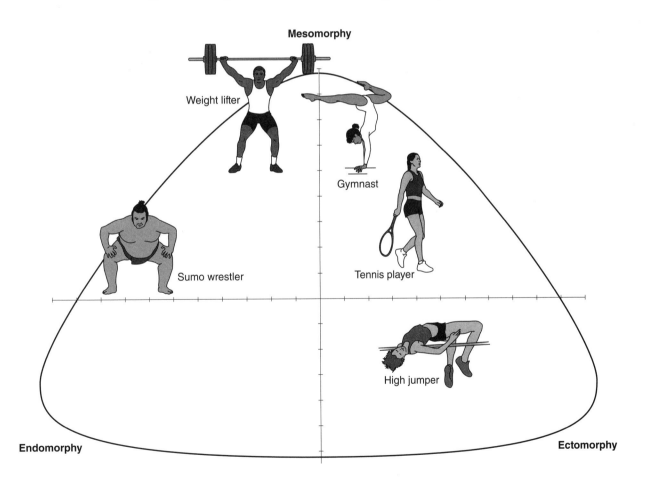

Figure 2.10 A somatograph is used to understand the degree of endomorphy, ectomorphy, and mesomorphy that an athlete's body possesses.

Table 2.5 Blood Markers for Monitoring Training

Marker	Uses in monitoring of training
Performance	
Creatine kinase	An indicator of muscle damage; rises during periods of intense training and returns to baseline with rest.
Cortisol	An indicator of stress; can be catabolic; known to reduce immune responses. Intense training may increase resting levels, and taper has been shown to decrease resting levels.
Testosterone Free testosterone (salivary)	Anabolic hormone that helps maintain muscle mass. Free testosterone is known to decline during periods of insufficient caloric intake or high levels of energy expenditure.
Glutamine: glutamate	Glutamine is a key amino acid in immune function and protein synthesis, and glutamate is a result of its metabolism. This ratio is used to assess tolerance to a training load. A significant decline below 3.58 in the ratio indicates intolerance to training.
Secretory immunoglobulin A (SIgA; salivary)	An indicator of specific immunity; decreases with prolonged training, which has been associated with increased risk for respiratory infection; monitor with changes in white blood cell count; monitor with changes in performance and health status.
White blood cells	A WBC count is a blood test to measure the number of white blood cells (WBCs). White blood cells help fight infections. They are also called leukocytes. There are five major types of white blood cells: basophils, eosinophils, lymphocytes, monocytes, and neutrophils.
Iron status • Serum ferritin • Serum iron • Total iron-binding capacity • Transferrin saturation • Hemoglobin • Hematocrit	The presence or absence of iron in the body greatly affects the ability to transport oxygen via hemoglobin and muscle enzyme activity. Low ferritin stores (stage 1 iron deficiency) do not allow for training adaptations to take place since iron is a necessary cofactor for optimal operation of aerobic metabolism. Reduced serum iron and a low transferrin saturation are evidence of stage 2 iron deficiency. Stage 3 iron deficiency is evidenced by a reduced hemoglobin concentration and hematocrit percentage and thus a reduced oxygen-carrying capacity. High-level training is dependent on oxygen transport and thus very reduced in stage 3 iron deficiency.
Health	
Lipid profile	Total cholesterol, HDL cholesterol (often called good cholesterol), LDL cholesterol (often called bad cholesterol), and triglycerides. Indicators of cardiovascular disease; HDL and LDL examined as a ratio. Influenced by type of fat in the diet, exercise, and genetics.
Metabolic panel	Indicates the status of the kidneys, liver, and electrolyte and acid–base balance as well as blood sugar and blood proteins. Abnormal results, and especially combinations of abnormal results, can indicate a problem that needs to be addressed.
Vitamin B_{12}	Important for the normal functioning of the brain and nervous system and the formation of red blood cells. It is involved in the energy metabolism of fatty acids as it relates to energy production.
Folate	Important in the synthesis and maintenance of new cells, especially red blood cells.
Vitamin D	Promotes the absorption of calcium and phosphorous; important in bone formation.

The monitoring of blood glucose and lactate during training can also provide insights about the benefit of fuel taken in during training and competition as well as the progression of training. The benefits of carbohydrate can be evaluated by monitoring blood glucose at rest, with and without carbohydrate in training, and should be tracked with subjective markers of hunger, thirst, concentration, and rate of perceived exertion. Lactate measured during training can indicate the reliance of energy metabolism on carbohydrate and can be tracked with workload to indicate shifts in fuel use with training. Decreases in lactate at a specific workload indicate a greater reliance on fat as a fuel source, and increases in lactate with an increase in maximal work capacity indicate an improved anaerobic capacity and reliance on carbohydrate.

Assessing Hydration Status

Proper hydration is key to ensuring quality training sessions. Monitoring body weight along with urine color (the first urine of the morning) and thirst is a simple means of determining whether hydration is adequate. Body weight when thirst is minimal and urine is of a pale yellow color (when held against a white background and compared to a urine color chart; see table 2.6) indicates a hydrated state. An additional measure that can be more accurate is urine-specific gravity (USG). This is a measure of excreted waste in the urine. When hydrated, the concentration is low, and when dehydrated the concentration is high. Table 2.7 can be used to quantify hydration status based on measures of urine-specific gravity.

The measurement of sweat rate can be a key factor in helping an athlete maintain a hydrated state and replace fluid lost during training. Total sweat loss can be measured with the following equation:

$$\text{sweat loss} = (\text{body weight before} - \text{body weight after}) + \text{amount of fluid intake} - \text{fluid lost in urination}$$

Body weight should be measured in dry clothing before and after the training session. A loss of 1 pound (.5 kg) is equal to 16 fluid ounces (fl oz) (480 ml). Sweat rate is then divided by the number of minutes or hours of training completed to give a measure of sweat loss per unit of time. Fluid consumption must be 1.5 times greater than the amount of fluid lost as body weight. An example of calculating sweat rate is provided in the sidebar.

Table 2.6 **Urine Color Guide**

Hydration status	Urine color
Very well hydrated	Hint of yellow
Well hydrated	Pale yellow
Minimal dehydration	Light yellow
Moderate dehydration	Yellow
Significant dehydration	Dark yellow
Very significant dehydration	Dark yellow/orange
Extreme dehydration	Dark orange/brown
Very extreme dehydration	Green/brown

Table 2.7 **Urine-Specific Gravity and Hydration Status**

Hydration status	USG
Well hydrated	<1.010
Minimal dehydration	1.010-1.020
Significant dehydration	1.020-1.030
Serious dehydration	>1.030

Example of Sweat Rate Calculation

Pretraining weight: 165 lb (75 kg)

Posttraining weight: 163 lb (74 kg)

Deficit = 2 lb (1 kg)

Fluid consumed: 16 fl oz (480 ml)

Training time: 90 minutes

Net fluid loss during training: 2 lb × 16 oz = 32 fl oz loss

Fluid replaced by drinking during training: 16 fl oz

Total fluid lost in sweat: 32 fl oz + 16 fl oz = 48 fl oz (1.5 L) in 90 minutes

Sweat rate: 32 fl oz (960 ml) per hour

Fluid needed to replace body-weight loss: 32 × 1.5 fl oz = 48 fl oz (1.5 L)

Conclusion

This chapter stimulates your thinking about the characteristics and energy system needs of different sports and provides suggestions for monitoring performance and key aspects of nutrition. In addition, it highlights the need for individuality when designing any program for an athlete—each program needs to take into account who the athlete is as a person and how the athlete gets to his or her own performance. Monitoring an athlete's progress and the effects of nutrition on training can greatly enhance the ability to characterize the athlete's needs. The more specific a nutrition or training program, the more effective it will be.

The first chapter showed you the scientific basis for creating a nutrition timeline. This chapter helps the timeline accommodate the athlete as an individual and the physical needs of the athlete's sport performance. The information you learn in the upcoming chapters will help you create your own unique timeline matched to the energy systems and performance areas that are necessary for the specific sport. The next step is to take the timeline and apply it to how an athlete views food.

Psychology and Sport Nutrition

Athletes are infamous for thinking of food as fuel for their bodies and sport, but this often becomes the main focus for athletes, and the art of listening to the body may be temporarily or permanently lost. This art is crucial because it provides the stepping stone from knowing and trusting the body to being able to get the most out of it and be successful in sport. Having the mental skills and strength to navigate nutrient timing is very important for athletes throughout the progression of sport. These skills should be developed at the very youngest age and should be continually refined throughout the sport development process. The mental approach to food plays an important role in achieving success in sport and life.

At the opposite end of the continuum are athletes who undergo training so they can justify the food and quantities they eat. However, it is preferable to approach nutrition and nutrient timing from the perspective of listening to the body and, more important, employing the principle of eating to train—appropriately feeding and hydrating the body in preparation for training sessions so the body is nutritionally prepared for the rigors of the physical training to come. Athletes who introduce proper nutrition before and after training sessions will receive the greatest positive adaptations to training.

Age and Nutrition

Paying attention to an athlete's age is extremely beneficial when implementing a nutrient timing plan because certain developmental stages require special nutrients, and these will change as the athlete matures. For example, the nutrient needs of an adolescent female who has begun menstruating will differ from those of an older female reaching menopause. Young athletes under the age of 20 are still developing their peak bone mass, and specific nutrients will be needed in higher amounts versus when they reach their 30s and 40s.

Measures of Age

chronological age –
The number of years an
athlete has been alive.

developmental age –
A measure of an athlete's
body size, psychological
function, or motor skills;
typically used by coaches
to determine progression
and level of readiness in
sport.

training age – A product
of the years the athlete
spends in a sport

Chronological, developmental, and training ages are often used when evaluating an athlete throughout the life cycle. **Chronological age** is measured by the number of years the athlete has been alive and is not typically a measure of physical performance. There are many chronologically older athletes who perform at high levels, and the opposite also holds true with some younger athletes. **Developmental age** is a measure of an athlete's body size, psychological function, or motor skills and is typically used by coaches to determine level of readiness in sport as well as to measure progress and the ability to continue to the next performance level (e.g., from national to international to Olympic competition). It is said that an athlete who has at least 10 years in a sport has progressed through the physical, mental, and nutritional (to a certain degree) stages that allow the next level of commitment to be implemented. Finally, **training age** is simply the number of years an athlete has been training for a specific event. This can often get confused with developmental age, but there are distinct differences. Training age is a product of the years the athlete spends in a sport, whereas developmental age accounts for physical and cognitive function and progression. This is important to take into account when approaching training because athletes will be in different stages based on their chronological, developmental, or training ages.

Stages of Development

Food plays an integral role from the very beginning to the very end of the life cycle. Young athletes should learn about food topics such as the different macronutrients and the importance of hydration when first introduced to sport. Throughout the growth and development process, nutrition beliefs are shaped and changed for better or worse. Sometimes an athlete deviates from his foundation knowledge of nutrition in search of "the next best thing" that will make him bigger, faster, and stronger. Athletes usually succumb to these temptations early in their development process or when pressure to perform is high. A solid belief system, high self-confidence, and strong discipline will assist athletes in determining the role of food in sport and will empower them to make decisions that will affect their current and future nutrition status. Role models, supportive teammates, coaches, and parents can be used to foster these psychological belief systems.

Stages of development can be useful for coaches when working with their athletes because different nutrition and educational messages can be implemented throughout an athlete's growth process. For example, teaching a younger or less experienced athlete about which foods contain carbohydrate, protein, and fat may be a good foundation step to teach from, while teaching specific nutrient timing strategies to enhance performance would be a more advanced progression as the athlete develops in his or her sport.

Knowledge of the stages of development can be particularly useful for helping parents of athletes learn the complexities associated with each stage. During the school-age years from ages 6 to 12, children often experience inadequacy and inferiority around peers, and there can be self-esteem challenges. Parents, while still important, become less authoritative, and youth look to their friends and networks for information. This can cause body-image challenges because comparisons will be made among youth, and the quest to fit in becomes the goal. Healthy eating practices that were emphasized early in this stage may begin to take a backseat to weight, and feelings of inadequacy about body composition become somewhat of a priority. For example, kids who grew up eating healthy foods may shift their focus to overall caloric intake because of the increasing body weight of their frames as they age; they may care less about healthy foods and possibly even restrict calories to account for weight gain.

The period of adolescence from 12 to 18 years of age introduces more instability. The athlete is neither a child nor an adult, and the struggle to find his or her own identity becomes the priority while moral issues and the struggle with an ever-changing social network become top stressors. It is during this time that healthy eating principles fall by the wayside, and body-image issues stemming from pressure to fit in come first. Body weight and body composition are important components of the balance between athletics and social groups. Young athletes are faced with difficult decisions surrounding food, performance, and the ability to remain in certain social networks. Athletes in this age group will put proper nutrition and nutrient timing at the bottom of their priority lists, usually because of increased social pressures from their peers. For example, athletes may eat a poor pregame meal because they are with their friends and want to fit in rather than think of the performance benefits of the pregame meal.

In the young adulthood stage, ages 18 to 35, intimacy through relationships becomes important, and depending on the level of the athlete, it may be difficult to navigate this time of life since finding a life partner becomes the focus. Weight may still be a dilemma during this courting phase of life, and self-esteem remains a delicate balance of internal gratification and external worth. Because athletes in this age group are faced with many stressors including social, career, and relationships, food can either be a deterrent or a positive model they develop, usually based on their social network. The feeling of invincibility that comes with being young is still apparent, and with this comes the thought process of being able to eat anything and "get by" with poor choices.

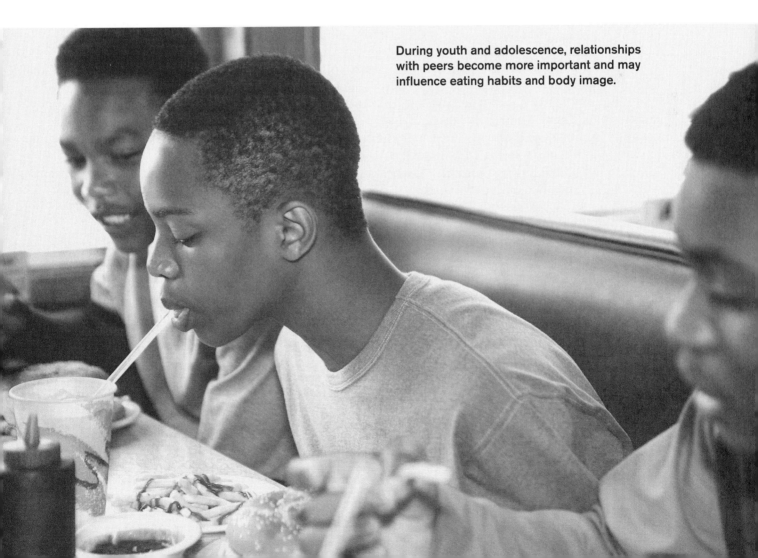

During youth and adolescence, relationships with peers become more important and may influence eating habits and body image.

In middle adulthood, ages 35 to 55, meaningful work and family become the focus, and the emphasis on self-confidence may take a backseat. Life goals change significantly as children leave the house, and reassessing life becomes a priority. If new meanings are not found, athletes can become stagnant and self-absorbed in their body image and nutrition. As the biology of aging takes hold, many physical changes are seen within the body, and because of the high stress of wanting to perform in a career and leading a family life, proper nutrition will be a secondary goal. It is not until after this stage in the life span that nutrition proves to be a higher priority as the athlete realizes the impact it can have on health in addition to performance.

Hunger and Eating Habits

As discussed in chapter 1, it is the input of the hypothalamus in the central nervous system that signals when food is needed to maintain body weight and support physiological processes. The hypothalamus can also drive what type of macronutrients the body desires to eat and when. This is something we refer to as instinctive eating. **Instinctive eating** is when we listen to our bodies in terms of when, what, and how much to eat and drink. By gaining an understanding of how our bodies tell us when and how much to eat, we can further maintain the blood glucose and insulin balance that helps optimize body composition and metabolism.

instinctive eating – Eating in response to physical hunger and cues from the body rather than out of habit.

We are all born instinctive eaters. You used to cry when you were hungry. This was your body's response to physical hunger cues; you listened to the cues and signaled to your parents to provide you with nutrients. You received nourishment and you were happy again, at least for the next few hours until physical hunger responses arose once again. Somewhere throughout the development process, instinctive eating knowledge is lost or forgotten, and athletes rely more on habitual hunger and forget about the cues their bodies are sending. The best example of habitual hunger is eating by the clock. If you eat at certain time intervals throughout the day, you are included in the habitual hunger group. You have lost touch with your internal body cues, and they need to be found again to incorporate food as an integral part of your sport development process.

Family history affects instinctive eating and the responses athletes have to food. Being raised in a "clean your plate before you leave the table" family structure is very different from meal times where the message is "leave food on your plate if you are not hungry." The first example teaches the body to hide its hunger—food is eaten because it is there, and because it is there, it must be eaten. The second example teaches the body to recognize the signs and patterns of fullness and enables the athlete to enjoy food while learning the different influences it has on the body at different times throughout the day. This example is what athletes should strive for, especially in this fast-paced lifestyle that encourages eating for the sake of fueling the body and not for the enjoyment and functionality of the food.

Habits also affect snacking behavior. People typically snack when they are hungry or nearing the 3-hour window between meals; however, an athlete must be aware of whether the hunger is habitual or physical. Habitual hunger is when an athlete "feels" hungry as a result of being accustomed to eating at a certain time. Physical hunger is the interaction between the brain, digestive system, and hormones of the body that sends a true pang of hunger, indicating that the body needs fueling. For many athletes this may seem strange, but it is necessary to reprogram the body into the instinctive eating patterns that were most likely overridden in youth. The end result is a far more frequent eating pattern (i.e., more snacks) that helps ensure stable blood glucose. This approach is dependent on the ability to plan in advance and is

Stress Eating

This athlete is a female distance runner who earned a collegiate scholarship at an NCAA Division I school. Moving away from home and needing to cook for herself, adjusting to a new coach, and learning to deal with a much harder level of coursework was a big change for her. In response to these stresses, she compensated by consuming foods that reminded her of home or made her feel good after a long day. These foods were high in sugar and fat, which only drove her to crave and eat more of them. Over time, her body weight steadily increased, and her performance began to decline because of a significant increase in body-fat mass.

The stress of poor performance and weight gain led this athlete to binge even more on unhealthy foods. An older athlete on the team recognized the stress this freshman was experiencing and how she was abusing food. The veteran had gone through the same thing in her freshman year, and she recommended that her young teammate seek help from the athletic department's nutritionist.

The first step for this athlete was to realize that food was being treated as an escape for issues she really needed to address in a direct manner. Second, the athlete had to learn respect for herself and her body. Once she accepted that food should be used to support her training and overall health, the athlete was able to begin catching herself when she used food to address stress instead of eating as a result of hunger or to support training.

To cope with the various stresses she was encountering, the athlete took the following steps:

1. Learned from the school sport nutritionist how to prepare meals that were quick to fix but full of flavor
2. Learned from the school sport nutritionist how to make better choices at the school cafeteria by reading the nutrition facts presented for each meal option
3. Created a timing system that was focused on optimizing food to support her training and competitions
4. Worked with a mediator to begin addressing the challenges she faced with her new coach
5. Sought the assistance of an academic advisor who could help her balance coursework with daily life

supported by research examining the effects of providing snacks to athletes between meals. As a result of the snacks, athletes unknowingly reduced the size of their meals. The athletes showed improvements in body composition, which led to improvements in anaerobic power and endurance.

When tuning in to instinctive eating at meals, it is not just the content of the meal that is important but also how much of the food is consumed and at what rate. If you are an athlete, it is important to monitor how full you are (by assessing hunger) and how satisfying the meal is. Once you are full, assuming you liked the meal, you should stop eating. This can best be done by using a scale such as the one depicted in figure 3.1.

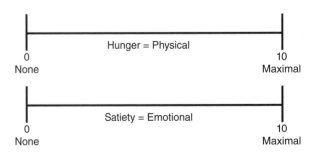

Figure 3.1 The hunger scale ranges from 0 (indicating no hunger) to 10 (indicating very high levels of hunger). The satiety scale ranges from 0 (indicating no satisfaction at all with the food or opportunities available to eat) to 10 (indicating a very high level of satisfaction with the food consumed).

Preparing for Nutrition Change

A change in a nutrition plan requires planning and preparation. In fact, defining the plan is one of the most important first steps when deciding to change a nutrition strategy. At the top of the list is realistic goal setting, which leads to forming the road map of change. Once the goals are identified and athletes know where they are going, it is important to identify the current state of mental readiness. Any change in nutrition requires a change in behavior and mental readiness to adopt new habits and actually implement them on a consistent basis. However, if an athlete is not ready to make a change in behavior, it is not appropriate to expect it or plan for it. Thus, knowing where athletes are beginning in the process is a key first step.

Stages of Behavioral Change

Stages of Change Model (SCM) – A model describing the mental steps people go through when preparing for and making a change in their lives.

Regarding behavior change, it is important to build a knowledge base using a popular psychological theory that assists in lifestyle and sport progression. James Prochaska and Carlo DiClemente developed the **Stages of Change Model (SCM)** in the late 1970s and early 1980s while studying how smokers tried to end their addiction. The rationale behind this model is that behavior change involves progression through many steps before the behavior is fully changed. These steps do not have a timeline since many athletes will progress at their own rate—and they should be allowed to without pressure from anyone. If you are planning a change in your nutrition plan, this model can help you understand why you have or have not been successful in the past and what steps you can implement in the future to get back on the right path and strive for optimal mental and physical performance.

In brief, the SCM is made up of five stages. Each stage has specific behavioral characteristics that help athletes determine their starting point and logical progression through the stages. Not all athletes begin at stage one. In fact, many enter at different stages, which is why it is important to determine which nutrition-specific behavior change stage an athlete is at in order to progress to the next one. If you are an athlete, the following are the stages of the SCM as they pertain to preparing for a nutrition change:

1. *Precontemplation.* In this stage, you do not acknowledge that there is a behavior to change, and you do not think seriously about changing. You are not interested in receiving any assistance from anyone, and you will defend your habit by not thinking it is a problem. You may be 10 pounds (4.5 kg) heavier than normal and not realize it is an issue, and when someone tries to tell you, you adamantly deny it. Simply put, you do not see yourself as having to change a behavior.

2. *Contemplation.* In this stage, you spend time thinking about changing your habit, but you do not act on it. It is purely a cognitive stage, where thinking about it is the extent of your progression. This stage is like riding a teeter-totter. You go up and down, weighing the pros and cons of changing but never land on solid ground long enough to make a change. You are more open to receiving information about changing your habit and will use educational methods to reflect on your thoughts and feelings about making the change.

3. *Preparation.* In this stage, you are committed to making a change, and you have fully embraced beginning the actual process by seeking out information to help you change your behavior. The focus is on small steps toward attaining your goal. Examples include identifying your meal timing and patterns throughout the day; determining whether stress, boredom, or emotions trigger eating higher-fat foods or larger quantities; and furthering your education by reading about these topics in order to build your knowledge level.

4. *Action.* In this stage, you exhibit high self-belief and confidence to change your behavior and be successful. Perhaps it includes shopping for healthier foods and learning how to interpret a nutrition facts label for performance information. The important thing is that you are actively involved in the change. Because you will rely more on your dedication, this stage can be volatile because the risk for relapse is high. However, you will typically form solutions to possible obstacles you will face from both yourself and others. Short-term rewards are used with great success. During this stage, you are willing to seek support from others, which can help prevent relapse. Develop a positive support system, those you know you can depend on in times of trouble, and use them. It will greatly assist you in progressing to the last and final stage.

5. *Maintenance.* The action stage may or may not take a while to complete, but once you get to the maintenance stage, you often have learned and developed the skills to stay here. Short bouts of relapse may happen, but for the most part, you have done the work to change your behavior, and you are working to maintain it. This stage involves being able to successfully avoid temptations. One characteristic of this stage is the ability to anticipate situations that may cause a relapse and have proven coping strategies and solutions ready and waiting.

Relapse

Although relapse is not a defined stage of progression in the SCM, it is important to mention because it is normal for athletes to regress as they learn about their bodies' nutrition needs and listen for their hunger cues. Some athletes fade in and out of relapse frequently, while others encounter only a few cases. It can be discouraging to enter into this stage. Some athletes feel a drop in their self-confidence after a relapse, but they should not. If you are an athlete, relapse is part of your journey of change, and it is healthy to navigate through this stage because there is much

Becoming educated and having a plan helps an athlete make confident nutrition choices.

you can learn about yourself and your ability to develop effective coping mechanisms that will get you back on track in a positive direction. Most athletes will cycle through some of the five stages of the SCM several times; this is not only completely normal but also expected. For you to continually add skills to your mental nutrition toolbox, you must learn more about yourself and how you approach food. Don't expect this to happen overnight or even within a few months. It will take commitment and dedication on your part, and you may not always be successful—and that is okay. Expect relapse. If you approach this with the idea that there will be hurdles and obstacles that will prevent you from being successful at times, then you will be more willing to allow these to come and go without sending you into a downward spiral where you are not progressing as quickly as you think you should.

If you slip on occasion, remember, you are not a bad person and you have not failed. This should not alter your self-confidence or belief that you can make a positive change and become a better person and athlete. You are merely allowing the natural progression of behavior change. One thing to note about relapse is that when it happens, be sure to not regress to the precontemplation or contemplation stage. It is extremely important to restart your process at the preparation, action, or even better, maintenance stage.

Goal Setting

Goal setting is very important for athletes since goals serve as markers of success and increase positive reinforcement through the immediate feedback provided during each training session. There are two major types of goals that athletes and coaches should understand: process and outcome.

Process goals are those that athletes have the most control over. Most of the emphasis and planning should focus on process goals, which provide incremental markers of progress and success along an athlete's developmental process in sport. These goals are conducive to positive behavior change because frequent results can be seen and used to facilitate positive progression. For example, process goals could include learning the difference between physical and habitual hunger or learning how to read a nutrition facts label for health and performance reasons. These well-defined short-term goals help athletes progress to their ultimate long-term goals.

In contrast, outcome goals are those over which athletes have little control. Athletes tend to set these goals more in the idealistic instead of realistic state of reference. Outcome goals are beneficial to have, but athletes and coaches should not place emphasis on their attainment. Rather, athletes should focus on attaining their process goals, which will lead to the end outcome goals. For example, an outcome goal could include something very general, such as learning how to fuel better before training sessions or competitions. It would be difficult to achieve this goal without setting realistic process goals that provide benchmarks for the progression.

Process goals can be a bit difficult to set without knowing how. The easiest way to approach setting process goals is to dissect the outcome goal into different stages. Process goals should provide continued progress toward the outcome goal without steering off course. If we use the example of learning how to fuel better before competitions, an athlete's process goals could include how to stay hydrated throughout the day, how to eat properly with the correct quality and quantity throughout the day, and what foods and beverages the athlete's body can tolerate well in the 1 to 2 hours before competitions. These process goals will lead to a successful outcome goal.

Using an Inside-Out Approach

Change must begin within an athlete first. The athlete must make character and intrinsic motivation the driving forces of change rather than allow her personality type (such as introvert or extrovert) to be the guiding force. It may be necessary to shift from an outside-in approach—where aesthetics and what others think matter most—to an inside-out approach of developing habits that support the behavior change and goal-setting process. Habits consist of skill (how to implement a plan to achieve a goal), desire (the motivation to move toward achieving a goal), and knowledge (what goals to set). Throughout the goal-setting process, athletes must relinquish dependence and move toward independence. Some goals will require the assistance of others, so to be truly successful in goal setting and achievement, interdependence is needed. The circle of trust with the experts who share their resources is formed and developed throughout the journey.

Once athletes learn the proper nutrition behaviors, they can be confident in their approach to food and what it does for them, and they will realize that the success of timing nutrient ingestion should be a priority for the effect it has on recovery-based performance enhancement. If you are an athlete, take the time to learn about your body's responses to certain foods and your hunger cues and feelings of fullness, and use this knowledge to pave your sport development path. Moving from dependence to independence to interdependence involves a series of steps.

We'll use the example of fostering a positive mind-set for weight loss. Most athletes, when they determine they are ready, simply jump into it with both feet without following the proper steps mentioned in the Stages of Change Model. It is crucial for athletes to approach a goal of weight loss very delicately since there is so much confusion on the topic and because there exists the possibility of not succeeding. Being proactive rather than reactive makes the process easier. An athlete who is trying to lose weight should use available resources and have a strong initiative to take charge of success (proactive) instead of focusing on a quantitative number of pounds or kilograms to lose and basing success on the scale (reactive). The athlete and coach should assess the situation from the beginning and continually make changes to the plan to promote successful attainment of the weight-loss goal, even when challenges present themselves. It is these challenges that will derail an athlete's goals if he reacts to them instead of being proactive and identifying solutions.

If you are an athlete, remember to focus your efforts on the journey and process goals instead of the larger outcome goal. Focus on the things you can influence, such as your self-confidence, your ability to make the right food choices, and the proper nutrient timing throughout the day to stabilize blood sugar. This is the proactive approach.

It is also important, in this example, to put yourself first. Some athletes try losing weight for someone else, but this decision must be internalized, and you must want it for your overall health, performance, and well-being. If you are an athlete trying to lose weight, make time for yourself, and set yourself up for success by surrounding yourself with a positive support system and identifying solutions to potential challenges that will arise. Reward yourself when you achieve your process goals. Acknowledge and celebrate these successes, although beware of how you celebrate. Food is often a reward mechanism, and in the example of weight loss, it is important to identify other non-food-related rewards when you move from step to step, such as new clothing or sports equipment or a special vacation. Finally, take time to enjoy the process, and remain in psychological, emotional, and spiritual balance without letting the process of change become too daunting.

The Road Map

There is something to be said about having a plan. Most coaches methodically plan training cycles and sessions to prepare their athletes for competition. Every intricate detail is accounted for—and with good reason. This lets the athletes know they are going into competition well prepared and with a plan of attack. The same holds true for nutrition. The more an athlete can take responsibility and be held accountable for nutrition planning, the more successful the athlete will be.

Taking the Step From Contemplation to Action

This athlete is a high school wrestler who has the potential to make the world junior championship team. At one time he was considered one of the most talented athletes at his weight class; however, over the past couple of years, he has not been able to perform at his best because of poor weight management in the off-season and the earliest part of the training year. He knows this is the main reason his energy is low on the mat during competition.

This past summer he was able to attend a training camp put on by one of his heroes—a wrestler who had multiple world titles and was considered by FILA to be one of the greatest who ever competed in the sport. One of the key secrets to success that this great athlete shared was that he learned to manage his body weight the right way, even in the off-season. It was something this young wrestler knew he should seriously consider if he was going to make it to the higher levels. After that camp, he was reminded every time he went to the grocery store what his hero had said at camp. He began to pick up items and just look at the nutrition contents on the back, often confused by claims made and discouraged because he could not understand what the nutrition facts labels actually meant.

That fall once the young wrestler was back in school, his cross country and wrestling coaches challenged him to get his weight under control so they could help guide him to an eventual spot on the world junior team. The fear of working with a nutritionist and what he would be asked to change—would it mean taking all the fun away from him and his friends when they went out?—was something that had to be addressed for this young athlete. The decision to take the leap into action was being hindered mostly by this one thing. Fortunately, his parents sought out a nutritionist who would work with him based on his own preferences and at a rate he could accept. Once the athlete realized the changes he needed to make were not quite as insurmountable as he had once envisioned, he moved forward at a very rapid pace.

For athletes, this means following the "eat to train, don't train to eat" mantra by ensuring their nutrient stores are at the necessary level before quality training sessions and competitions as well as not rewarding themselves with food. Athletes who do not have access to food and beverages after training sessions should put their postworkout or competition food in a cooler. For weight-class athletes, developing a plan for making weight in advance will help prevent the last-minute rush of weight cutting the day before competition, which may have a negative effect on performance. When traveling nationally or internationally, athletes and coaches need to identify food locations and sources at the destination where the food is safe to eat. If this is not possible, athletes should take their food with them along with the necessary equipment to cook it. This is the type of planning that is required to navigate a successful journey. Using a nutrition road map makes the journey much easier because athletes and coaches can see where they want to end—they simply need to develop a plan to get there.

Education

The most confident athletes are those who are physically, mentally, and nutritionally prepared. When an athlete has knowledge and experience about food and the role it plays in sport, it is easier to be confident about making nutrition decisions. To improve self-confidence, athletes need to develop nutrition foundation skills during the early stages of nutrition planning. These concepts include what nutrients are included in which foods, how to read a nutrition facts label for health and performance, how to understand the ingredients list on food labels, how to create a shopping list and navigate the grocery store successfully, and how to understand the difference between wholesome and refined or processed foods. Learning more about the body is also crucial throughout the development process and will serve as a springboard in making the correct nutrition choices at the right time. Identifying when the body is biologically hungry versus habitually hungry is the first step in improving self-awareness and confidence. Additionally, recognizing why athletes choose a certain food at a certain time will help identify emotional eating behaviors and prevent overeating.

Sticking to the Plan

Athletes who are committed, consistent, and persistent in carrying out their nutrition plans will benefit the most. Roadblocks will surface throughout the development process that continually test an athlete's commitment level and ability to adapt to change. Being an athlete is synonymous with adaptation, whether physical, mental, or nutritional. The solutions an athlete and coach develop to these challenges along with the athlete's responses to obstacles will shape the athlete's persona and athletic endeavors.

Of course it would be unfair not to mention discipline and sacrifice. Athletes live and breathe these on a daily basis. The same amount of discipline is needed in nutrition planning and implementation as is required in completing training sessions and competing at the highest level possible. Discipline in doing that last set of intervals, spending a few extra minutes after practice to develop their skills, and being a student of their sport will take athletes farther. The same holds true with nutrition. Being disciplined when it comes to making the right food choices and implementing a nutrient timing program will make a tremendous difference in an athlete's progression through life and sport.

Of course, most of this mental nutrition training should begin with the end in mind. What are you trying to achieve in the long term, and what path will you carve to get there? If you are an athlete, think about what you want to accomplish physically, and then work backwards and pay special attention to your mind-set about nutrition, your nutrition knowledge, the mental challenges you face, and the continued education you need in order to successfully adopt new nutrition behaviors along the way. These continual improvements to your mind and the role nutrition plays will guide you to success. There will be times when you face obstacles, sometimes appearing to have no solutions. However, this is part of normal behavior change and the mental adaptation response to learning new skills.

If you are a coach, you can assist your athletes by helping them identify the challenges that will come between them and their goals. Offer possible solutions to these challenges and help the athlete understand that there are many ways to overcome barriers and obstacles. Helping the athlete to create a plan with specific, measurable action items will help in this process.

Conclusion

Embracing the concepts outlined in this chapter, such as realistic goal setting to develop a solid plan of action and incorporating the behavior change principles associated with the psychological Stages of Change Model, will assist athletes in their quest to improve their nutrition habits. Athletes who identify their support systems and progress from being dependent to independent to interdependent will find it much easier to achieve their large outcome goals through successful navigation of the smaller process goals that make up the journey of behavior change.

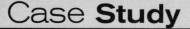

Weight Loss and Body Composition Changes

This case study describes a female collegiate soccer player with a goal of losing weight and decreasing body fat to improve performance. Her main position is striker (forward). She was just coming off of her competitive season and had a month off from structured practice before resuming conditioning. The holidays would be a challenge as her off-season and return to pre-season conditioning would fall around the holiday season.

BACKGROUND OF SPECIFIC ISSUES RELATIVE TO NUTRITION

In the past, the athlete had not periodized her nutrition to match her training seasons and thus was not successful at reducing her body weight and body fat percentage. She found herself eating too much food in the preseason and thus was not at a good competition weight for her season. Because she did not want to negatively affect performance, she did not try to actively lose weight during her competition season, instead saving that goal for her off-season.

NUTRITION GOAL

Her main goal is to lose weight to improve her running speed. Although she did not set a goal for body fat percentage, she does want to focus more on losing body fat than lean muscle mass.

NUTRITION PLAN

The first step for this athlete in her journey of weight and body-fat loss was identifying her emotional connection to food and the reasons she chose certain foods at certain times throughout the day. This athlete was accustomed to using food as fuel and not approaching food from a positive mind-set.

The athlete started a food (and exercise) log so she could record what, when, and why she ate throughout the day, which helped identify the main challenges that were holding her back. Her support group analyzed the types of food she ate throughout the day along with her timing preferences, but preliminary work focused on highlighting the reasons behind her food timing and food choices. During the three days she kept the food and training log, there were noticeable times of eating because of emotions and habit rather than hunger. These were easy to identify because the column "why" in the food log included the words "boredom," "tired," and "stressed." She also identified times she ate because of cravings.

The mind-set of using food only as fuel can be detrimental in the beginning phases of weight loss. This athlete in particular needed to change her thought patterns—from the "food as fuel" mind-set she was used to during her competitive season to the "when is my body hungry?" mind-set that is a foundation of nutrition during the off-season. This simple shift allowed her to recognize her internal body cues to hunger and satiety, which would help with weight and body-fat loss.

After identifying her main initial challenge as her emotional connection to food, she learned about the components of biological hunger, stabilizing blood sugar, and satiety. The primary goal was to teach her to recognize her body's cues for biological hunger and identify the specific differences between these and emotional or habitual hunger. Biological hunger can be identified by physical signs such as stomach pangs or mental signs such as a decrease in cognitive function and concentration. The latter is due to the fact that the brain operates predominantly on glucose, and when levels are low, concentration and cognitive abilities decline. Because normal blood glucose levels ebb and flow about every 3 hours, her support group asked her to begin identifying the physical and mental signs of biological hunger and eat only when she was biologically hungry for five days. Her energy expenditure was fairly low because she was in the off-season; therefore, if she could not identify her hunger before she was really hungry, it would not affect her exercise performance. At most, she was exercising for 45 to 60 minutes per day of combined cardiovascular and light strength training exercises, so she did not require a higher number of calories or a greater volume of food to sustain a higher level of training.

Throughout the five days, she continued to keep her food log indicating what, when, and why she ate, and she began to learn when her body needed food for the maintenance of normal body processes and when she ate because food was there or because she was stressed or bored. After these five days, she was able to easily see what situations and scenarios were emotional triggers for eating. Once she identified the triggers, she developed solutions so she would be armed with the knowledge of what to do when faced with these challenges. For example, this athlete went home to her parents during holiday break and was faced with many high-calorie snack foods that she would normally overconsume out of emotional hunger. Typically, she felt obligated to eat because someone made the snacks or because the holidays are often seen as a time to eat less healthily. The solution was for her to provide positive feedback to the person and express thanks for the snack foods but politely decline eating the food because she was not hungry at the time. This was difficult for her at first because she was a "people pleaser," but she practiced it at home before going to social holiday gatherings.

Stabilizing blood sugar was her first nutrition intervention because significant blood sugar fluctuations will lead to instances of uncontrollable eating, overeating, and feeling out of control. She followed a nutrition plan that focused on eating a source of lean protein, healthy fat, and a fruit or vegetable at every feeding time with minimal consumption (if any) of whole grains and starches. The combination of the lean protein, healthy fat, and fiber found in the fruit and vegetables improved her satiety factor (kept her fuller longer), so she did not experience the blood sugar "crashes" that normally lead to emotional eating. Additionally, the significant reduction in whole grains removed unnecessary calories from her nutrition plan during the off-season.

Any athlete's daily nutrition program should be based on the statement "simple is sustainable." This athlete's first step to support this mantra was to develop a list of foods that she enjoyed and would eat. The foods were then categorized into lean protein and healthy fat, fruits and vegetables, whole grains and healthier starches, and "misses." This final category is very important to identify and allow in an athlete's nutrition plan because it supports positive behavior change progression. The misses category includes any foods that do not fit in the other categories and usually encompasses foods that are eaten sporadically as indulgences (desserts, snacks, and so on). As a homework assignment, she drew four columns on a piece of paper, creating a form similar to figure 3.2 (p. 54), with each column titled with one of the food categories just described. Next, she wrote down the foods she enjoyed, regularly ate, and would like to eat in each category. It was important that she list ample foods in the lean protein and healthy fat and the fruits and vegetables columns, since those foods would primarily make up her daily nutrition plan. The next step was for her to bring her food lists to life, so to speak. She identified three or four different food combinations that she could implement for breakfast, lunch, dinner, and snacks, all based on the foods she listed. There were no strange foods to buy or recipes to follow. It was all based on what she enjoyed eating.

The nutrients she chose to put together would act to support her hunger and keep her fuller longer. Her goals included (1) to eat only when she was biologically hungry, (2) to pick a food from the lean protein and healthy fat column and a food from the fruits and vegetables column 90 percent of the time and eat them together at meals and snacks, (3) to increase her consumption of lean protein and healthy fat by 25 to 50 percent of what she would normally eat, and (4) to allow herself to have misses 10 percent of the time. That is, she would trust herself and be confident that she could and should allow herself to eat foods that did not fit into one of the main columns, because this is part of the process of developing a positive relationship with food.

Food Lists for a Nutrition Plan

**Protein and Fat, Fruits and Vegetables,
and Grains and Starches = 90% of Total Food Intake**

Lean protein and healthy fat	Fruits and vegetables	Whole grains and healthier starches

Misses (10% of Total Food Intake)

Figure 3.2   A form like this one can help athletes identify familiar foods they like for their nutrition plans.
From K. Austin and B. Seebohar, 2011, *Performance nutrition: Applying the science of nutrient timing* (Champaign, IL: Human Kinetics).

Keep in mind that this type of nutrition plan should be introduced to athletes only during the off-season or early part of preseason training as it will provide only enough energy to support a lower training load. When training load increases, athletes should be more flexible with the types and amounts of food they eat.

Reshaping this athlete's paradigm of thinking about nutrition and approaching it from a perspective of biological versus emotional hunger was not a quick process. It rarely is because this is a behavior change. Over the off-season and into the first month of preseason training, she was able to improve her ability to recognize her biological hunger cues, and she felt more in charge of her eating patterns and decisions. This led to just over 6 pounds (3 kg) of weight loss, and she returned to preseason conditioning with a lighter body, which enabled her to train more efficiently.

FOUR

Functionality of Foods

To create an optimal nutrition plan, it is necessary to understand the role of a food in promoting recovery and adaptations to training. A functional food is one that has a defined benefit to health and performance. Typically, there is at least one component in the food that has a specific function and will produce a positive physical effect beyond just the nutrition content of the food. In principle, the type of food that is taken in along the nutrient timeline should promote goals such as improving the energy systems at rest and in training, promoting muscle recovery, controlling appetite, optimizing body composition, and supplying essential nutrients as well as provide the satisfaction that should come from enjoying food.

There are external and internal signals that control when and what a person will eat. External factors include the environment (e.g., cold versus hot weather), social habits (e.g., always having soda when eating out with friends), or even finances (food affordability). Internally, the sensations of hunger, fullness, satiety, or discontent will determine the frequency and size of meals. Becoming aware of the external and internal signals that influence food intake is the first step to ensuring that the function of the food eaten is appropriate. **Macronutrients** are the primary nutrients found in the body and diet: carbohydrate, fat, and protein. Each of the macronutrients plays a role in assisting with the internal cues that help control food intake. If you understand the functions of each macronutrient, what you or your athlete eats suddenly takes on more meaning. The food can be utilized to serve a purpose.

macronutrients – The primary nutrients (carbohydrate, fat, and protein) found in the body and diet.

Digestion of the Macronutrients

Understanding the **digestion** and **absorption** of the macronutrients can greatly aid in determining how appropriate they are in an athlete's nutrition timeline. The functionality of a food is very dependent on how quickly it can be digested and absorbed by the body. The digestion of all the macronutrients begins in the mouth. Digestion in the mouth is started by enzymes that are responsible for breaking down complex carbohydrates. Chewing assists in digestion by breaking food down into smaller particles, and this process is further driven by the stomach. As food moves into the stomach, the macronutrients are separated, and from this point there is a significant difference as to how they will finish being digested and absorbed by the body.

digestion – The process used by the body to break down food into substances that can be absorbed.

absorption – The uptake of nutrients by the tissues of the body.

Carbohydrate moves from the stomach to the small intestine, where all forms of carbohydrate (except for fiber) are absorbed. The smaller the food particle becomes, the quicker it can be emptied into the small intestine. More enzymes then act to break the pieces down into monosaccharides (the simplest form of carbohydrate), which can be absorbed by capillaries in the intestine's walls. As monosaccharides enter the blood, they are transported to the liver for further breakdown and then either enter the blood as **glucose** or become stored as glycogen in the liver or muscle.

glucose – The element of carbohydrate that the body uses as its primary fuel source.

Not all of the carbohydrate content in foods can be digested and absorbed. The amount that is not absorbed may be a result of the form the food comes in, the amount and type of fiber present, or the type of starch. Large amounts of indigestible carbohydrate in the form of fiber, starches, or milk sugars can lead to increased gas production or other disturbances such as cramping and diarrhea. The fiber that cannot be digested by the body plays an important role in maintaining a healthy intestine and the ability to transport broken-down food in a timely manner. Fiber also influences the glycemic response of a food by slowing the rate at which it is digested, and as a result fiber can aid in maintaining stable blood glucose levels and optimizing body composition.

amino acid – A building block for protein.

Protein is predominantly digested in the stomach. Stomach acid separates protein into smaller and smaller strands until it can be broken down into the basic units of **amino acids.** The amino acids then travel to the small intestine, where they are absorbed into the blood for delivery to the body's cells. The liver is the key regulator of the body's amino acid pool and will direct what happens with incoming amino acids. In some instances, protein will serve as an energy source and aid in muscle repair, and at other it times it will just be stored in the amino acid pool of the body until it is needed for making additional proteins.

Fat is the slowest of the macronutrients in terms of breakdown. As the stomach begins to break down carbohydrate and protein, fat sits on top because the fluids of the stomach can do little to digest it. From the stomach, fat enters the small intestine, where bile and pancreatic juices break it down into smaller pieces and move it into the bloodstream. It will then be either used as a fuel or stored as an energy reserve.

Understanding Carbohydrate

The average athlete can store approximately 1,600 to 1,800 calories from carbohydrate in the muscles, liver, and blood. Carbohydrate balance is regulated very well in situations of energy balance. When carbohydrate is consumed it stimulates storage (glycogen) and **oxidation** (glucose) as well as inhibits fat oxidation. Glucose that is not stored as glycogen is burned almost in equal balance to the amount that is consumed.

oxidation – The rate of energy release from the food consumed.

The simplest way to evaluate carbohydrate is to honestly ask how good it might be for the body. What purpose does it serve an athlete? Carbohydrate foods that are rich in vitamins and minerals and provide more than just empty calories should be the primary source in the diet. This can best be categorized by viewing carbohydrate as wholesome versus refined. Wholesome carbohydrate foods have the greatest nutrition value and contain only naturally occurring sugars. This includes fruits, vegetables, and whole grains, which contain vitamins, minerals, and fiber to aid overall body health. This form of carbohydrate helps ensure a strong immune system and contains **antioxidants** that take care of damage done during training and competition. Refined and highly processed carbohydrate foods such as candy, white bread, cereals high in sugar, and other high-sugar products such as cakes and cookies are primarily composed by adding sugar to the carbohydrate that is already present and as a result these foods are not very nutritious.

antioxidant – Any substance that can prevent or delay the breakdown of a product in the body.

Alcohol and Performance

Alcohol is frequently associated with sporting events, whether it is related to an athlete's celebrating a win or just a part of the culture that comes with a sport. Alcohol is a form of carbohydrate; however, unlike other forms of carbohydrate that enhance performance, alcohol typically decreases an athlete's performance through its effects on concentration and athletic skills. Alcohol inhibits metabolism and also interferes with the body's ability to properly utilize vitamins and minerals. Underneath the concept of nutrient timing, the time and place for any significant amount of alcohol is during the off-season or when celebrating a key performance. Large amounts of alcohol can inhibit restoration of muscle glycogen stores, and thus energy reserves for recovery after training and competition are not available. As a result, the athlete may be at an increased risk for injury. High concentrations of alcohol in the body can also dehydrate an athlete, and this further increases the risk for injury and heat strain during training and competition. In addition, for many athletes alcohol increases caloric intake and can result in weight gain.

The key to alcohol is to understand the appropriate time and amount that should sensibly be consumed. When an athlete is in training and trying to achieve high-performance goals (one of which might require a lean physique), regular consumption of more than two glasses of alcohol per week may significantly impair this process. It is important for athletes to replace all of their carbohydrate stores and other necessary nutrients required for health and performance before consuming alcohol, even just one glass. Athletes should think about their performance goals and then consider how to best accommodate alcohol into their performance lifestyle.

An athlete's diet will often contain both types of carbohydrate; refined sugars can greatly aid in making food palatable and can be used to aid in recovery immediately after exercise. The key is to ensure that refined carbohydrate does not replace the wholesome carbohydrate necessary to ensure a healthy body that can perform without breaking down.

Carbohydrates are typically classified as being simple or complex. Simple carbohydrates can be broken up into three groups: monosaccharides, disaccharides, and oligosaccharides. Monosaccharides include the sugars glucose, fructose, and galactose. They are all made up of only one sugar molecule and are the easiest and fastest to digest. Monosaccharides are considered to be the primary energy unit for the body's cells, and most important, glucose is the primary energy source of the central nervous system. Disaccharides include sucrose, lactose, and maltose. These each contain two monosaccharides and thus are not as easily digested. Oligosaccharides are made up of 3 to 10 monosaccharides and include maltodextrins, corn syrup, and high-fructose corn syrup. This form of carbohydrate is typically manufactured and takes longer to digest. Complex carbohydrates are polysaccharides that are long, complex chains of sugars that require a more complex digestion process than simple carbohydrates. They include foods that are known as starches and those that contain a significant amount of fiber. This includes oat bran breads and cereals; yogurts; and even fruits and vegetables such as cucumbers, cabbage, onions, plums, strawberries, and oranges. Complex carbohydrates cannot always be fully digested.

It was once thought that simple sugars were the "bad" form of carbohydrate and complex carbohydrates were the "good" form. Now that the glycemic response of foods is understood, this is no longer the case. Research has shown that the glycemic response of both simple and complex carbohydrates can vary greatly and is dependent on a person's own metabolism. As a result, an athlete must look at carbohydrate foods based on quality and determine which ones are wholesome and which ones are poor in nutrition value.

The glycemic response is the measure of a foods or drinks ability to raise blood glucose. Figure 4.1 shows the glycemic response pattern in healthy adults. This response is highly dependent on the structure of the carbohydrate ingested; the amount of protein, fat, and fiber in the food or drink; the amount of food consumed; the content and time of any previous food or drink; and the digestion and absorption process for each person's own metabolism. The glycemic response is determined based on the **glycemic index (GI)** and **glycemic load (GL).**

glycemic index (GI) – A ranking system that classifies carbohydrate foods based on how they affect blood glucose levels.

glycemic load (GL) – A ranking system that takes into account the GI of a food as well as the portion size consumed to determine the effects on blood glucose.

The GI is a measure of how quickly 50 grams of a food or drink's carbohydrates are converted into glucose and how this affects blood glucose over a 2-hour period. Glycemic load is defined by the amount of carbohydrate in a serving of the food or drink ingested. As a result, the GL takes into account the volume of food or drink consumed and thus is more appropriate. A GL of 20 or more is high, a GL of 11 to 19 is medium, and a GL of 10 or less is low. The GL for a single serving of food (100 grams) can be calculated by the quantity of its carbohydrate content (in grams) multiplied by its GI divided by 100.

Glycemic load = carbohydrate content (g) $\times$ (glycemic index / 100)

For example, a 100-gram serving of watermelon with a GI of 72 and a carbohydrate content of 5 grams can be calculated as follows:

$$5 \text{ g} \times (72 / 100) = 3.6$$

The GL is 3.6.

In the same sense, foods with very different GIs can provide the same GL. A food with a GI of 100 and a carbohydrate content of 10 grams has a GL of 10 (10 $\times$ 1 = 10), while a food with 100 grams of carbohydrate and a GI of 10 also has a GL of 10 (100 $\times$ .1 = 10).

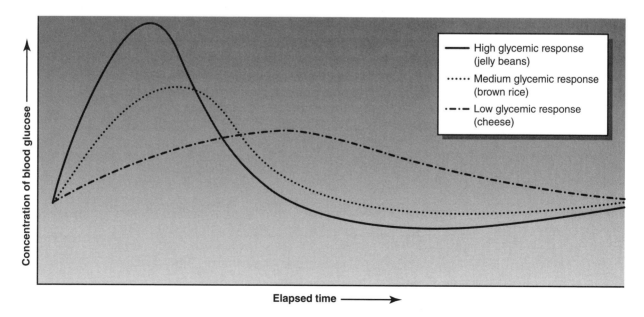

Figure 4.1 Increase in plasma glucose levels from foods with high, moderate, and low glycemic indexes (GIs).

Although being able to calculate the GL can be of benefit, it is the ability to read a food label for its total content that is most important. Additionally, this can highlight how critical the other components of a food (fat, protein, and fiber) are in determining the quality of the food being consumed. Figure 4.2 shows examples of food labels classified based on the glycemic response. The function of a food or drink along the timeline of nutrient ingestion should be to produce stable blood glucose levels throughout the day, which helps the body minimize large fluctuations in energy intake and output. The goal should be for an athlete to achieve a response similar to that demonstrated by foods that produce a low glycemic response.

Understanding Protein

Proteins are composed of a large number of amino acids. There are two types of amino acids: essential and nonessential. Essential amino acids

Nutrition Facts

Serving Size 8 fl oz (240ml)

Amount Per Serving

Calories 50 | Calories from Fat 0

% Daily Value*

Total Fat 0 g	0%
Saturated Fat 0 g	0%
Trans Fat	
Cholesterol 0 mg	0%
Sodium 110 mg	1%
Total Carbohydrate 114 g	5%
Dietary Fiber 0 g	0%
Sugars 14 g	
Protein 0 g	

Vitamin A	0%	Vitamin C	0%
Calcium	0%	Iron	0%

* Percent Daily Values are based on a 2,000 calorie diet. Your daily values may be higher or lower depending on your calorie needs.

a

Nutrition Facts

Serving Size 1 bottle

Amount Per Serving

Calories 250 | Calories from Fat 50

% Daily Value*

Total Fat 5 g	8%
Saturated Fat 1.5 g	8%
Trans Fat 0 g	
Cholesterol 10mg	3%
Sodium 180 mg	8%
Total Carbohydrate 34 g	11%
Dietary Fiber 0 g	1%
Sugars 31 g	
Protein 14 g	

Vitamin A	45%	Vitamin C	50%
Calcium	50%	Iron	25%

* Percent Daily Values are based on a 2,000 calorie diet. Your daily values may be higher or lower depending on your calorie needs.

b

Nutrition Facts

Serving Size 1 packet: 1.98 oz. (56.12 g)

Servings per Container 1

Calories 200 | Calories from Fat 5

Amount per serving | % Daily Value*

Total Fat 1 g	2%
Saturated Fat 1 g	5%
Trans Fat 0 g	
Cholesterol 0 mg	0%
Sodium 240 mg	10%
Potassium 140mg	4%
Total Carbohydrate 33 g	11%
Dietary Fiber 3 g	12%
Sugars 1 g	
Protein 13 g	23%

Vitamin A	0%	Vitamin C	100%
Calcium	1%	Iron	11%

* Percent Daily Values (DV) are based on a 2,000 calorie diet.

c

Figure 4.2 Nutrition labels from foods with (*a*) high glycemic response, (*b*) medium glycemic response, and (*c*) low glycemic response.

are those that must be consumed in the diet or else the body will become deficient, and nonessential amino acids are those that can be made by the body. Amino acids build and repair body tissues, become hormones or facilitate the action of hormones, maintain fluid and electrolyte balance, promote the immune system, aid in the transportation of other nutrients within the blood, balance the body's systems, and can serve as an energy source both during exercise and at rest. Protein can also help control appetite and increase the energy necessary to digest a meal. As the protein content of a meal increases, so does the use of protein as an energy source; however, this is highly dependent on the availability of carbohydrate and fat.

Protein in the diet can come from a wide range of foods including meat, fish, dairy, soy, legumes, nuts, grains, and vegetables. The quality of protein derived from these food sources is dependent on the amino acid content and the digestibility of the protein. Proteins derived from foods such as meat, dairy, and whole grains are considered to be complete proteins because they contain all the essential amino acids and have approximately 95 percent digestibility. Plant proteins from foods such as legumes and vegetables are usually classified as incomplete proteins since no single plant food contains all the essential amino acids, and their digestibility reaches only up to 85 percent.

Proteins have also been classified as fast and slow. This primarily centers on how protein is used in building muscle mass and promoting the desired glycemic response. The focus of this classification is on casein and whey proteins, which are both derived from milk. Approximately 80 percent of whole milk's protein is casein, and the other 20 percent is whey. Whey protein is absorbed by the body much more rapidly than protein from other food sources. For this reason, this fast protein is often used as a supplement. Since whey protein is fast to digest, it can provide large increases in amino acids to the body; however, this is short lived. If timed appropriately with training, this can translate into a transient increase in muscle synthesis. Whey also has higher levels of leucine, a potent amino acid that stimulates protein synthesis.

Casein on the other hand is considered a slow protein because of the time it takes to digest and be absorbed, as well as its ability to slow the emptying of foods from the intestines. Casein is relatively insoluble and forms structures called micelles that increase solubility in water. This is the basis for why casein has a slower rate of digestion and results in a slow and steady release of amino acids into circulation. However, a steady supply of amino acids may help prevent protein breakdown for a longer period of time. As a result the body will maintain a protein balance that is more positive. Since whey rapidly increases protein synthesis and casein and other slow proteins block protein breakdown, a combination of both may be ideal.

The goal with nutrient timing is to utilize the fast and slow properties of a protein to help facilitate the desired glycemic response. When a high glycemic response is desired, a fast protein such as whey must be utilized so that digestion time does not slow down the ability of glucose to enter the bloodstream. Conversely, when a low to moderate glycemic response is desired, slow proteins such as those found in casein, soy products, and lean meats can assist in creating this response.

Protein has been shown to create training adaptations and potentially a metabolic advantage in weight loss. Athletes have been documented as easily meeting the recommended protein requirements for the general population because of an increased energy intake needed to support training. Although some research has begun to examine protein needs for athletes, there is no conclusive evidence regarding how much protein is required for optimizing training adaptations. What is known about protein is that the type and timing of its ingestion will work with other macronutrients to influence the response of the muscle to training.

A wide range of protein intake (1.2 g/kg to 3.0 g/kg of body weight) has been suggested for athletes depending on the type, intensity, and duration of training an athlete undertakes. It is important that the range of intake for any one macronutrient energy source always ensures that health is maintained and that adequate intakes of the other essential nutrients are possible. Under generally accepted U.S. nutrition recommendations, as much as 35 percent of energy can be derived from protein while still maintaining the recommended intake for the macronutrients of carbohydrate and fat. See chapter 6 for more information on dietary guidelines that should be met by any nutrition plan, including Recommended Dietary Allowances (RDA), Dietary Reference Intakes (DRI), and Acceptable Macronutrient Distribution Ranges (AMDR).

Understanding Fat

On average, the body stores upward of 80,000 calories as fat. Dietary fat can play many important roles in the function of the human body. Although it is a significant source of energy during rest and exercise, it also provides fatty acids that are essential for making hormones and driving functions such as blood clotting, absorption of key vitamins (A, D, E, and K), the body's immune response, the regulation of heart rate, blood pressure, and the function of all the body's tissues. It also cannot be ignored that fat helps make food taste good! A large range (.8 g/kg to 3.0 g/kg of body weight) of daily fat requirements has been recommended for athletes depending on the sport, position, and duration and intensity of training. Obtaining the proper amounts and types of fat can have a positive impact on both health and performance.

Foods can contain both visible and invisible fats. Visible fats are those foods such as oils, butter, creams, and additional condiments that can easily be seen when added to food. Typically almost 100 percent of the calories found in these foods come from fat. Invisible fats are those that already exist in foods or that are put into foods and cannot be seen. This includes the fat that may be in a piece of meat, fish, or cheese and even the fat that comes from avocados and nuts. To determine that these fats are in the food, you need to read the contents of the food label. Invisible fats are the major source of fat in most people's diets.

Dietary fat is found primarily in the form of triglycerides, followed by phospholipids and sterols (cholesterol). Triglycerides are made up of three fatty acids and a glycerol backbone. Fat can be classified as either saturated or unsaturated, and the differences in structure can have a significant impact on health. Saturated fats are usually solid at room temperature (e.g., butter), and their fatty acids are saturated with hydrogen, which can have a negative impact on heart function. These types of fats are found in animal products such as fatty meats, creams, whole milk, butter, and cheese. They can also be found in snack foods such as cookies and chips and oils such as palm, coconut, and palm kernel. Unsaturated fats (e.g., olive oil) are usually liquid at room temperature and have one or more fatty acids that are unsaturated by hydrogen.

Unsaturated fats have three subgroups: monounsaturated, polyunsaturated, and trans fats. Trans fats have been hardened by hydrogenation, making them even worse for health than saturated fats. They can also cause an increase in the levels of "bad" cholesterol (low-density lipoproteins, or LDLs) and lower the levels of "good" cholesterol (high-density lipoproteins, or HDLs). These types of fat are commonly found in fried foods; snack foods such as doughnuts, crackers, and cookies; and processed foods and margarine. Trans fats are often not listed on food labels, so athletes should pay particular attention to the ingredients, looking specifically for *partially hydrogenated oil* in the list. This is an indicator that trans fats are present in the food.

Conversely, mono- and polyunsaturated fats can have a positive impact on heart function by improving the ratio of good and bad cholesterol and keeping blood vessel function healthy. Monounsaturated fats are beneficial to health and blood lipids, and most food sources also contain vitamin E, which acts like an antioxidant and is important in sport. These types of fat, in general, are more health promoting and can be found in foods such as olives, avocados, walnuts, salmon, trout, and oils including soybean, corn, safflower, canola, sunflower, and olive.

Polyunsaturated fats include the omega-3 and omega-6 fatty acids, which cannot be made by the body's cells and must be consumed in the diet. Omega-6 fats are converted to arachadonic acid in the body. Omega-3 fats are converted to eicosapentaenoic acid (EPA) and docosahexaenoic acid (DHA). The less EPA and DHA is formed, the greater risk of increased inflammation in the body. Because athletes already experience a high degree of internal inflammation due to training, it is important to reduce inflammation as much as possible.

The ratio of omega-6 to omega-3 fatty acids is important and ideally is 3:1. A low ratio is preferred because the omega-6 fatty acids compete with the omega-3 fatty acids for the same enzymes so that they can be broken down. In the Western diet, the ratio typically ranges from 10:1 up to levels of 30:1 since omega-6 fatty acids are commonly available in vegetable oils. Since Western diets include such a high level of omega-6 fats compared with omega-3 fats, very little omega-3 fats are converted into the healthy EPA and DHA compounds. As a result, it is important to cook with oils and consume foods rich in omega-3. Since it is not overly abundant in food, it may be necessary to supplement the diet with omega-3 to optimize the body's cholesterol levels.

Omega-3 fatty acids can help significantly in the regulation of blood pressure and cholesterol. They can also assist in recovery from training by decreasing inflammation, improving growth hormone levels, and assisting with a healthy immune system. They can additionally improve oxygen delivery to the body by decreasing blood thickness and as a result improving aerobic metabolism, potentially leading to an improved ability to utilize fat as a fuel source. Omega-3 fats have also been shown to increase the body's internal antioxidant enzymes, increase sensitivity to insulin, and prevent hyperglycemia. Overall, athletes should place an emphasis on increasing omega-3 fat intake in their nutrition program and decreasing saturated and trans fat intake while lowering omega-6 fats to a moderate amount so omega-3 conversion to EPA and DHA is better supported. Tilting the balance of omega-6 to omega-3 intake can easily be done by lowering the use of oils such as corn, safflower, sunflower, cottonseed, and soybean and substituting with olive and canola oils. Athletes should pay particular attention to nutrition ingredient labels to identify these oils in foods. Consuming enough omega-3 fats in the daily nutrition plan should be a goal for all athletes and can be achieved by selecting from the following list:

- Anchovies
- Flaxseed
- Flaxseed oil
- Mackerel
- Herring
- Salmon
- Tofu
- Walnuts
- Walnut oil
- Soybeans
- Navy beans
- Kidney beans
- Pumpkin seeds
- Canola oil
- Trout

Analyzing Nutrition Labels

FOOD 1

Would this food have a high, low, or medium glycemic response? Why? How quickly would it be digested?

> This food would have a high glycemic response. It would be digested very quickly because of the sugar in the source of carbohydrate and the fact that there is little fat or fiber content in the product.

What types of fat are present in this food? How healthy are these fats?

> The food does not have any fat content.

What is the source of protein? Is it a slow or fast protein?

> The protein most likely would be broken down quickly since the label indicates that it is whey protein.

Nutrition Facts
Serving Size 2 scoops (91 g) (makes 12 fl oz)

Amount Per Serving

Calories 320	Calories from Fat 0

	% Daily Value*
Total Fat 0 g	0%
Cholesterol 0 mg	0%
Total Carbohydrate 60 g	20%
(100% from Dextrose)	
Sugars 60 g	
Protein 20 g	40%
(from Whey Protein Isolate, Milk Protein Isolate, Hydrolyzed Whey Protein)	

Vitamin A	50%	•	Vitamin C	670%
Vitamin D	50%	•	Calcium	50%
Sodium	15%	•	Potassium	6%

* Percent Daily Values are based on a 2,000 calorie diet. Your daily values may be higher or lower depending on your calorie needs.

FOOD 2

Would this food have a high, low, or medium glycemic response? Why? How quickly would it be digested?

> This food would have a low glycemic response. It would be digested very slowly because of the minimal sugar content along with a very low ratio of carbohydrate to protein and fat. In addition, a large part of the carbohydrate source is fiber.

What types of fat are present in this food? How healthy are these fats?

> This food product has a moderate fat content in relation to the carbohydrate and protein levels; however, the fat is not saturated and thus it appears to be a healthy fat.

What is the source of protein? Is it a slow or fast protein?

> We do not know the type of protein provided. However, protein lowers the glycemic response and so would help to further reduce the already low glycemic response of this food.

Nutrition Facts
Serving Size 1/4 cup

Amount Per Serving

Calories 130	Calories from Fat 40

	% Daily Value*
Total Fat 4 g	6%
Saturated Fat 0.5 g	2%
Trans Fat	
Cholesterol 0 mg	0%
Sodium 150 mg	6%
Total Carbohydrate 10 g	3%
Dietary Fiber 8 g	32%
Sugars 1 g	
Protein 14 g	28%

Vitamin C	2%	•	Calcium	4%
Iron	10%	•		

* Percent Daily Values are based on a 2,000 calorie diet. Your daily values may be higher or lower depending on your calorie needs.

Fuel Oxidation

Understanding a food's release of energy can assist in determining the function of the food. Oxidation is the rate of energy release from food consumed. The body can utilize all the macronutrients for oxidation. The macronutrient utilized is dependent on what type of fuel the body has learned to use at rest and during exercise. In chapter 2, this is described as the respiratory exchange ratio (RER). The RER at rest and during exercise is reflective of the relative percentage of fat and carbohydrate used to supply the energy needed to perform at a set workload.

The interpretation of the RER at rest and during exercise indicates how well a person can utilize fat and carbohydrate, which can be very important in altering body composition and weight. Most important is the interpretation at rest for nonendurance athletes, as the majority of energy expended throughout the day is through resting metabolism. Protein oxidation cannot easily be measured by this method; however, protein utilization by the body at rest and during exercise has been well documented and will be discussed in this section. When thinking about the function of a food and training goals, it is important to consider what type of fuel utilization an athlete should improve.

Fuel Oxidation at Rest

Fat is ideally the fuel source for oxidation at rest. At rest, fat should provide anywhere between 80 and 100 percent of energy demands, while carbohydrate and protein will provide between 5 and 20 percent and 2 and 5 percent, respectively. The body's ability to utilize fat at rest is dependent on the type of foods taken in and their glycemic response as well as whether or not the body has performed exercise that teaches it how to utilize fat as a fuel source. Foods that create a moderate to high glycemic response result in an increased reliance on carbohydrate as a fuel source at rest. This is further promoted when high-glycemic carbohydrate foods are consumed immediately before and during exercise. When food is consumed that provides a low glycemic response, the body must utilize a greater amount of fat as a fuel source to help supply the energy required to sustain life and perform exercise. Eating the right balance of macronutrients will elicit positive physiological adaptations on a cellular level that will favor more fat oxidation at rest and during exercise.

Improving fat oxidation at rest requires providing the right amounts of the macronutrients at any one time point. It is known that intake of carbohydrate results in an increased oxidation of glucose and that fat oxidation is decreased, whether at rest or during exercise. As a result, it is important not to consume too much carbohydrate all at once and to consume carbohydrate foods that take time to digest so that carbohydrate moves into the bloodstream much more slowly. By doing this, carbohydrate will not impede fat oxidation at rest.

In the same sense, protein intake results in a proportional increase of this macronutrient for oxidation and a reduced oxidation of fat. Protein oxidation at rest has been shown to be directly proportionate to the volume consumed; however, as with all energy sources, significant excess is stored as fat. This further highlights the importance of the type and volume of food as well as the frequency of eating. A large amount of protein should not be taken in at any one point in time. An athlete does not want protein oxidation to inhibit the body's use of fat as a fuel source.

Fat is not oxidized at rest when glucose is too high; this is why large meals that contain too much carbohydrate or protein can directly and indirectly lead to fat storage.

In a direct manner, excess carbohydrate in the diet will get stored as fat when glycogen stores are saturated and insulin spikes to deal with the high levels of glucose in the blood that result from large intakes of carbohydrate. In addition, carbohydrate and protein can indirectly contribute to body-fat storage by serving as a fuel for oxidation, and as a result, any excess energy consumed as fat will be stored by the body. This will also inhibit fat use at rest until the carbohydrate has been stored and the protein has been oxidized. The key to optimizing fat use at rest is to control the portion of foods eaten and to minimize large elevations in glucose, thus allowing the body to rely on fat at rest.

The ability to utilize fat as a fuel source while at rest is an important part of maintaining good body composition. The amount of energy used to sustain the body at rest accounts for the majority of energy expended throughout the day (the only exception being endurance athletes who perform a very high volume of training on a daily basis). The primary reason for fat accumulation is the excess intake of carbohydrate, protein, and fat in relation to the rate at which they can be oxidized and the energy expended in the day. For an athlete who wants to reduce body-fat levels, fat utilization while at rest cannot be inhibited, and energy can be provided only at the rate at which it is being used. Consuming foods that promote the utilization of fat as a fuel source helps reduce the body-fat levels that are present and aids in preventing further fat accumulation.

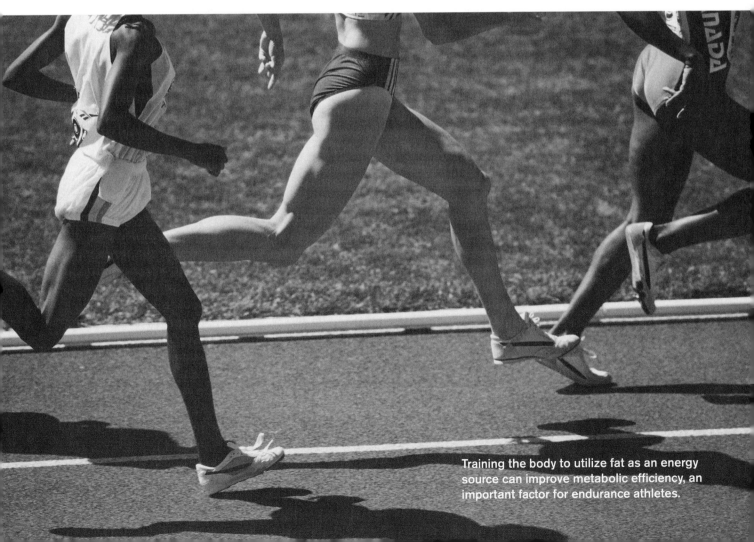

Training the body to utilize fat as an energy source can improve metabolic efficiency, an important factor for endurance athletes.

Fat and Carbohydrate Oxidation During Exercise

The oxidation of fat and carbohydrate during exercise is dependent on the body's ability to use fat as a fuel source and the rate of carbohydrate consumption. Low- to moderate-intensity exercise relies on the greatest proportion of energy from fat, unless carbohydrate is consumed immediately before or during the exercise bout. Consuming carbohydrate during these training sessions teaches the body to rely on it; however, the goal is usually to teach the body to use fat as a fuel source and promote fat oxidation. Ensuring as much fat utilization as possible during low- to moderate-intensity exercise requires little or no intake of carbohydrate.

The human body has an almost endless storage of fat that can provide energy for hours of training. Although this sounds very promising, many athletes do not understand that eating certain foods and following a well-planned training program without consuming carbohydrate can teach the body to become more efficient at using fat as energy. Learning to utilize the abundant fat stores that the body holds can translate into less of a reliance on the body's carbohydrate stores during exercise. This in itself has the potential to increase time to exhaustion and prevent the early onset of fatigue by protecting glycogen stores.

Interestingly, some research indicates that at lower work intensities, carbohydrate supplementation decreases gene regulation for fat oxidation. In other words, taking in more carbohydrate during training may actually decrease your body's ability to use fat as energy. Although carbohydrates are very important, the body cannot depend on them to provide all the energy needed during longer and higher-intensity training sessions or competitions because it's impossible to completely replenish the carbohydrate stores that are being expended. This is why it is important to become more metabolically efficient and teach the body to use more of its stored fat.

These concepts highlight a key factor in the timing of nutrient ingestion. The timing and volume of carbohydrate consumption before and during exercise must match the objectives of training. When the objective of training is to improve the body's ability to utilize fat as a fuel source and improve oxidative capacity, carbohydrate should not be consumed in the window immediately before or during training. This trains the body to utilize fat as a fuel source while at rest, and together with an energy deficit from training, this can significantly improve body composition.

During moderate to intense exercise, carbohydrate oxidation increases and can occur at approximately 1.0 to 1.5 grams per minute depending on muscle glycogen stores and the availability and type of carbohydrate taken in during the exercise bout. During competition and in key high-intensity training sessions, the consumption of carbohydrate is important to ensure that glycogen does not become depleted, as fat cannot generate energy quickly enough to meet the demands placed on the body during high-intensity activities. During exercise, protein can also be used through aerobic metabolism to generate energy for anywhere between 5 and 15 percent of the total energy cost; however, when carbohydrate and muscle fat stores are readily available, protein is used very little by the body because of the time necessary to convert it into usable energy. Greater amounts of protein are typically oxidized as the duration and intensity of the exercise bout increases and the availability of carbohydrate and muscle fat stores decreases.

Using the Functional Foods

The manipulation of carbohydrate, protein, and fat tends to have one of the following purposes: (1) controlling appetite, (2) optimizing body composition, (3) aiding muscle recovery, and (4) enhancing performance during training or competition. The goal is to utilize each of the macronutrients for a key function that is related to achieving nutrition and performance goals. If you understand the function a food has, you can determine how to best time the type of food utilized to restore the body's energy systems and assist in manipulating body weight and composition.

Appetite Control

Carbohydrate, protein, and fat all differ in their mechanisms for controlling appetite. Understanding each macronutrient's function in controlling appetite underlines why each should be a part of a consumed meal. The complex carbohydrate in a meal helps control appetite and size of the meal by sending the initial signal to the brain (via the blood) that food is being consumed and by satisfying receptors in the gut that determine fullness. Protein controls appetite by releasing satisfaction signals to the gut and most importantly the brain. Protein controls hunger longer than any other macronutrient, perhaps because of its ability to act on the hypothalamus, the area in the brain that signals food intake. The use of protein in conjunction with fiber to control the glycemic response of a meal is a key function of its ability to aid in body-weight management.

Fat can help satiety in two very different ways. When the fat content of a meal is eaten and reaches the intestine, it slows the emptying of carbohydrates, proteins, and fluid, thus making the gut feel fuller longer. Fat also helps food taste good and as a result provides satisfaction when you start eating. The fat content in a meal must be carefully planned, and it is recommended that it rarely be greater than 20 percent of the meal's composition. When a meal is too high in fat, the pleasure signal that is sent to the brain often stimulates a drive to consume more of the high-fat food. Additionally, fat in and of itself does not promote a feeling of fullness, and thus a meal that is too high in fat often results in greater portions of food eaten at one time, until a person feels full. Thus, while fat does have a role in a meal's composition, it must be used sparingly and in conjunction with the right type of carbohydrate and protein.

Body Composition

It has been previously mentioned that body composition is optimized through steady blood glucose levels and that large rises and drops in energy intake can lead to an increased development of fat mass. As a result, it is important that foods be combined to deliver a slow and steady supply of glucose to the blood. Under this scenario, carbohydrate should rarely be consumed without some form of protein, fat, or both. The combination of carbohydrate (with a high fiber content), slow-release protein, water, and a small amount of fat as a meal or snack will result in a slow rate of digestion. Foods that meet these criteria include stir-frys made with lean meats; salad with grilled chicken or fish; and low-fat dairy products combined with whole-grain cereals or high-fiber fruits such as berries, apples, bananas, and prunes and other high-fiber food items such as beans and lentils. The body's blood glucose level will remain very stable, and the majority of the food will be oxidized as fuel to keep the body running throughout the day.

Muscle Recovery

Muscle recovery is best facilitated via the window after training and at night when sleeping. Immediately after training, carbohydrate and protein rapidly provide glucose and amino acids that will restore muscle glycogen and aid in the synthesis of muscle that was broken down during the training session. Under this scenario, carbohydrates that can easily be absorbed are necessary and will most likely come in the form of monosaccharides disaccharides and high molecular weight starches. Athletes should consume protein or amino acids that can be quickly absorbed, such as those in whey protein or an essential amino acid supplement.

Sleep is considered one of the best methods of recovery, and thus the quality of sleep an athlete gets is very important. Consuming carbohydrate with a high glycemic response in combination with protein that has the amino acid tryptophan readily available (dairy, meats, nuts, soy) can potentially decrease the amount of time necessary to fall asleep and may also increase quality of sleep. If the type of protein ingested provides a slow release throughout the night, such as casein, which is found in milk and other dairy products, the available protein can potentially act with growth hormone to optimize the synthesis and repair of muscle.

Performance Strategies

The ingestion of fuel to optimize training and competition is dependent on the goals of the training session. As a result, it is necessary to develop strategies for supplying the working muscles with the optimal fuel. Fat, carbohydrate, and protein each serve as the primary functional fuel in specific types of training sessions. The goal is to manipulate the volume of these macronutrients to create a training adaptation.

Fat can be used strategically to enhance performance when consumed at the appropriate times. The use of fat at rest and as a fuel during exercise can lead to improved body composition and potentially performance. Increased fat usage during exercise

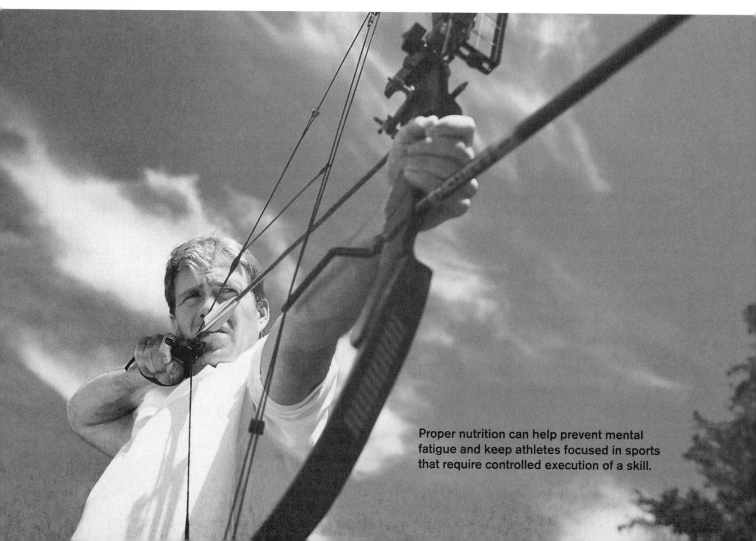

Proper nutrition can help prevent mental fatigue and keep athletes focused in sports that require controlled execution of a skill.

can result in lower levels of lactic acid production, and lower levels of fat mass can improve an athlete's economy of movement.

There are several approaches to strategically improve fat usage in the body. The first and most common is the use of training to either promote fat utilization or reduce the volume of fat in the body. Aerobic or low-intensity training increases the number of mitochondria and enzymes associated with fat metabolism, which will increase the ability of the body to use fat as a fuel source. Anaerobic or high-intensity training is the most efficient means of fat loss because of the greater overall energy expenditure. As exercise intensity increases, the volume of fat being burned also increases. As a result, the type of training performed should be dependent on the goal. For many athletes, the goal is for both adaptations to occur, and thus a program of mixed exercise intensities is best.

A second means of improving fat utilization is using diet composition to deprive the body of carbohydrates; simply removing high-glycemic carbohydrate from the diet before and during training can teach the body to rely on fat as a fuel source. Lastly, the use of medium-chain triglycerides (MCTs) in the form of anoil (typically sold as a supplement) that can be rapidly absorbed before training may have the ability to move fats from their storage sites and enhance their use during training. At rest, MCTs may even have the potential to improve fat usage or create a greater diet-induced thermogenesis, both of which could lead to improved body composition. These concepts are covered in more detail in chapter 6, which discusses fat as a fuel source and the timing of fat ingestion to optimize its role in the diet.

Carbohydrate ingestion can enhance performance during intermittent or continuous exercise of 45 minutes or longer. This can be for a training session or in competition. When carbohydrate is used in training, it supplies readily available fuel for the anaerobic energy system; thus, its functional role as a fuel during training is often to increase anaerobic capacity. It can also fuel athletes who must sustain a high functional power for long periods of time, and by ensuring a quality training session, carbohydrate enhances muscular endurance. Blood glucose also serves as the primary fuel for the brain. The central nervous system helps control mood, focus, and important factors in sport such as reaction time and contraction of the muscles. If blood glucose runs low during bouts of intense exercise, this will result in a depressed function of the central nervous system, and in turn mental and muscle function will be impaired.

Protein as a functional fuel can serve two primary roles when consumed before an exercise session. The first is to supply amino acids for building muscle during resistance training. Second, protein can serve as an energy source during exercise through its breakdown and conversion to glucose. This primarily occurs when there is insufficient carbohydrate available and there is a high demand for glucose (e.g., during a high-intensity training session).

Essential amino acids can also be used as a functional tool to stabilize glucose and the brain's level of various amino acids. Mental fatigue will directly lead to muscle fatigue because the brain controls the ability of the muscle to contract. In sports that require the controlled execution of a skill or rapid decision making for a prolonged period of time, essential amino acids may be beneficial for minimizing mental fatigue.

Mental fatigue is related to the amino acid tryptophan. Tryptophan aids in making serotonin in the brain. The role of serotonin is to induce relaxation, which can often cause a person to feel tired. During prolonged exercise bouts and periods of focus, an increase in tryptophan crossing the blood–brain barrier and raising serotonin levels can occur for a number of reasons. The amino acid tyrosine acts on the central nervous system to minimize the effects of serotonin and can functionally minimize mental fatigue and thus muscular fatigue. Essential amino acids also have the potential to enhance focus and concentration by assisting in the control of blood glucose. The branched-chain amino acids (leucine, isoleucine, and valine) can all improve the interaction of glucose with insulin and thus stabilize blood glucose levels. They also minimize the ability of tryptophan to cross the blood–brain barrier. In events of long duration, these essential amino acids can ensure that surges in blood glucose do not occur when the consumption of fluids with carbohydrate and foodstuffs may be necessary to maintain hydration and manage hunger. They may also be able to improve central nervous system status.

Another way to utilize the macronutrients from a performance standpoint is to classify them based on whether they are high- or low-residue foods, depending on how much waste is left in the large intestine after digestion. The residue of a food depends primarily on how much fiber content the food has but also takes into account the amount of nonlean protein and fat in the food. Typically, a person should have a high-residue diet that contains significant amounts of fiber. There are situations in sport, however, when **low-residue foods** are important to ensure competitive success. This includes weight cutting for weight-classified sports; competing in endurance events where gastrointestinal distress might be high; and exercising in hot environments where foods might not be able to "sit" in the stomach, predominantly because it does not feel good to the athlete. A list of foods associated with high versus low residues can be found in table 4.1.

low-residue foods – Foods that are designed to reduce volume in the stomach and typically contain less than 10 grams of fiber in the daily diet.

Conclusion

The goal of this chapter is to understand the basics of carbohydrate, protein, and fat in terms of structure and function in the body. The concept of timing nutrient ingestion is about not just the "when" but also the "what" in the food you eat. Understanding the function of a food further supports why just counting calories is not enough for an athlete. A food must serve a purpose to the training plan. The goal of the next three chapters is to dive further into how an athlete can functionally utilize the different macronutrients under specific circumstances to optimize training adaptations.

Table 4.1 **Low- and High-Residue Foods**

Food group	Serving size examples	Low residue	High residue
Breads and starches	1 slice bread 1/2 cup cooked cereal 1/3 cup pasta or rice 6 crackers	**Bread:** White bread Rolls Biscuits Muffins Crackers Pancakes Waffles	**Bread:** Whole grain Stone-ground cracked wheat Pumpernickel Dark rye Whole-grain crackers Whole-grain muffins Whole-grain cereals Corn bread Corn muffins
		Cereals: Corn Flakes Rice Krispies Special K Puffed rice Cream of Rice Cream of Wheat Grits Farina	**Cereals:** Oatmeal Any product made with seeds, nuts, coconut, bran, or dried fruits
		Other starches: White or sweet potato, no skin White rice Pasta (low fiber)	**Other starches:** Whole-wheat pasta Brown rice Buckwheat Millet
Fruits	1/2 cup canned Medium piece of fresh fruit	Strained fruit juice Canned or cooked fruits (no skins or seeds) Ripe banana Soft cantaloupe or honeydew Apricots Nectarines Papaya Peach Plum Watermelon Grapes Applesauce Fruit cocktail	Juice with pulp Prune juice Berries Figs Prunes Dried fruit

(continued)

Table 4.1 *(continued)*

Food group	Serving size examples	Low residue	High residue
Vegetables	1/2 cup cooked 1/2 cup raw without seeds 1 cup vegetable juice	**Cooked:** All but those listed as high residue **Raw:** Cucumber Green pepper Onions Romaine lettuce Tomatoes Zucchini **Juice:** Tomato Carrot	Lima beans Green peas Corn Broccoli Parsnips Juice with pulp
Dairy products	1 cup yogurt or milk 1 oz (30 g) cheese	Milk Yogurt Cheese	Products with seeds and nuts
Meats and protein substitutes	1 oz (30 g) cooked	Tender well-cooked meats Fish Poultry Eggs Tofu Creamy peanut butter	Tough meats with gristle Legumes (beans, peas, lentils) Crunchy peanut butter
Fats	1 tsp regular or 1 tbsp reduced fat	Butter Oils Salad dressing Mayonnaise Cream Gravies Whipped cream Creamy peanut butter	Seeds Nuts Olives Coconuts Poppyseed dressing Crunchy peanut butter
Miscellaneous		Plain cakes, cookies, pastries, and pies Sherbet Gelatin Sugar Hard candy Condiments Coffee, tea	Anything made with whole grains, bran, seeds, nuts, coconut, or dried fruit Candy made with chocolate or nuts Chocolate syrup

Functional Foods for Body Composition

This athlete is a female collegiate long jumper and 100-meter sprinter. She is 20 years of age and has been participating in the sport for 8 years. This year the athlete is looking to set personal records in her events. In the next 2 years, she hopes to become an NCAA All-American.

The long jump and 100-meter sprint are both events in track and field. The long jump requires athletes to combine speed, strength, and flexibility as they attempt to leap as far as possible from the takeoff point. There are four main components of the long jump: the approach, the last two strides, the takeoff and action in the air, and the landing. The two fundamentals of success are the speed obtained in the approach and a high leap off the board. Speed is such a critical factor of the approach that most long jumpers are also very good sprinters. Competition typically consists of three jumps of which the best score counts. In high-level competitions, there is a preliminary and final round.

The 100 meters is an explosive power event much like the long jump. It also requires speed, strength, and flexibility as well as very quick reaction time for getting out of the blocks. Because athletes must move their center of mass at very high velocities, it is important that they maintain a low level of body fat so that efficiency is as optimal as possible.

BACKGROUND OF SPECIFIC ISSUES RELATIVE TO NUTRITION

Over spring break, the athlete attended a camp for jumpers and had her body composition analyzed. Her sum of 7 was at the top of the range for elite jumpers. The coach suggested that she work on improving her body composition, which should in turn improve speed and power production. He also recommended that she monitor her performance using a 30-meter acceleration test, the sprint fatigue test, and the amount of weight she could clean for a three-repetition maximum. This would allow her to gauge the effectiveness of the nutrition program she might implement to improve her body composition.

A review of the athlete's nutrition practices showed that she had a very consistent eating pattern and consumed an adequate number of fruits and vegetables. She had also been taught the importance of hydration for recovery and helping to ensure that she did not increase her chances of pulling a muscle. Her weakest area was that she had a tendency to eat too many energy-dense carbohydrate foods, which she believed her body craved as a result of her hard training days. To study for school effectively, she satisfied these cravings so she could focus and not be distracted.

NUTRITION GOAL

Knowing that focus is important for her study habits and that reducing food intake could have a negative effect on her in-season performance, her support team recommended that she wait until after her regeneration period to begin working on her nutrition program. The goal during the season and throughout the regeneration period was to monitor feelings of hunger and satiety. The hope was that this would help control the volume of sweets and starchy carbohydrate foods she was consuming.

NUTRITION PLAN

After the two-week regeneration period, she did another baseline body composition test as well as the recommended performance testing. The nutritionist determined that the athlete could potentially reduce fat mass by 5 pounds (2.3 kg) and that this was feasible over the next three months. Training would occur in three-week blocks followed by a recovery week. A program of intermittent high-intensity exercise was introduced four days of the week that rotated soccer, tennis, basketball, and kickboxing for 1 to 2 hours. The other two days of the week were used to maintain speed and power through strength and conditioning.

In addition, she identified three ways to improve her nutrition intake:

1. Identify healthy sweet treats that were lower in calories.
2. Consume only half of the sweets that she craved, and reduce the volume of starches she consumed at meals.
3. Attend a yoga-based meditation class that would teach her other ways of coping with stress and also improve her flexibility.

The nutritionist also increased protein consumption to one-third of meal composition and asked her to increase the number of fruits and vegetables she consumed by 25 percent. The timelines show typical daily food intake for this athlete before and after the nutrition program. The monitoring of performance testing and body composition occurred at the end of every three-week period. Over the summer months, she was able to lose the 5 pounds of fat mass, gain 2 pounds (.9 kg) of muscle mass, and improve her true speed while decreasing her rate of fatigue.

Timeline

Typical Daily Meals Before Nutrition Program
- **Prerun snack:** Banana with peanut butter
- **Postrun snack:** High-glycemic carbohydrate, protein drink
- **Breakfast:** Cereal, whole milk
- **Lunch:** Potato with chili, fruit
- **Snack:** Chips and salsa
- **Dinner:** Hamburger, fries, salad
- **After-dinner snack:** Toast with jam
- **Late-night snack:** Peanut M&Ms

Timeline

Sample Daily Meal Plan to Improve Body Composition
- **Prerun snack:** Whole-grain bagel, low-fat cream cheese, banana
- **Postrun snack:** Low-glycemic carbohydrate, protein recovery beverage and fruit, dark chocolate
- **Breakfast:** Oatmeal, skim milk, hazelnuts, agave, raisins
- **Lunch:** Whole-grain homemade barbecue chicken and vegetable pizza
- **Snack:** Mango and cottage cheese
- **Dinner:** Cumin-rubbed salmon, marinated vegetables, polenta
- **After-dinner snack:** Spiced applesauce

As she reentered the school year, she was asked to touch base with the athletic department's sport psychologist and life counselor to identify additional ways to keep stress levels down. In addition, she would continue participating in yoga through classes offered at the school recreation center. She would touch base with the nutritionist once monthly for a body composition check and to hold her accountable. She also made the following nutrition commitments to help her avoid falling back into her old habits:

1. Use hunger and satiety to gauge how much sweet and starchy foods I can consume.
2. Create a list of favorite snacks and meals that meet my nutrition requirements.
3. Prepare or purchase my healthy sweet treats in advance.

Timing Fluid Intake

Water is the most important nutrient for the human body. It makes up approximately 60 percent of an average person's body weight and can fluctuate between 45 and 75 percent based on age and body composition. The amount of water in an athlete's body depends on many factors including age, sex, body composition, and overall body size. Water is stored in different locations in the body including fat (10 percent), bone (22 percent), muscle (70 to 80 percent), and blood plasma (90 percent); significant reductions of fluid in these areas can have a negative effect on performance and cognitive function due to dehydration. The goal for athletes most of the time is to remain in a well-hydrated state considering their sport's requirements in order to maintain good health and optimal performance.

Trained athletes can have relatively high total body water values because of their higher lean mass, and glycogen loading can sometimes increase total body water in some athletes. This is an important consideration for some athletes who compete in weight-class or acrobatic sports such as wrestling, weightlifting, boxing, gymnastics, taekwondo, and figure skating because the precompetition hydration and carbohydrate strategy should be very individualized to meet the weight-control demands of each of these sports while ensuring an optimal state of hydration before competition.

Optimal absorption of fluids is important for athletes before, during, and after a training session. When a fluid is equal to the **osmolality** of the body, it is termed **isotonic.** A **hypotonic fluid** is a fluid that is less than the osmolality of the body and is emptied from the stomach more quickly, while a **hypertonic fluid** is a solution that is greater than the normal body's osmolality and is emptied from the stomach more slowly. The faster a fluid empties from the stomach, the more advantageous it is to athletes because this reduces the risk of gastrointestinal distress and lets fluids reach the cells quickly to keep the body in a **euhydrated** state. This means better and faster fluid delivery to the cells and muscles to be used for training and competition.

During exercise, an increase in body core temperature will increase skin blood flow and the loss of fluid and electrolytes through sweat. Evaporation is the primary method of heat loss during exercise and can be fairly substantial in warm and dry environments. Sweat rate is highly individual to each athlete and depends on characteristics such as body weight, genetic predisposition, metabolic efficiency, and heat acclimatization. Because of this, sweat and electrolyte losses range greatly among athletes in the same sport and within different sports and positions, as discussed later in the chapter.

osmolality – A measure of the concentration of substances such as sodium, chloride, urea, potassium, and glucose in the blood.

isotonic fluid – A fluid equal to the osmolality of the body.

hypotonic fluid – A fluid that is less than the osmolality of the body.

hypertonic fluid – A fluid that is greater than the osmolality of the body.

euhydrated – Having an adequate amount of water to meets the body's physiological demands.

Testing Hydration Status

Assessing an athlete's hydration status is a very important marker during training. Even a slight decrease in body weight due to fluid loss can lead to a performance decrease. Ideally, hydration testing should be accurate enough to detect total body water changes of about 2 percent of body weight (the level of fluid loss shown to affect exercise performance). Practical tests to monitor hydration include urine-specific gravity, use of a urine color chart, and body weight.

A simple test done in the laboratory, urine-specific gravity (USG), can be easily taken into the field to test an athlete's daily hydration status. A hand-held refractometer is needed along with a urine cup and pipette. An athlete simply provides a small amount of urine, and a few drops are placed in the refractometer for analysis. Within a few seconds, a USG number is provided that can be used to educate athletes on their daily hydration status. Refer to table 2.7 on page 39 for USG reference numbers corresponding to different hydration states. Cost of this equipment varies, but it is an accurate way to quantify an athlete's hydration state. Additionally, it is extremely easy to transport and perform this test anywhere the athlete is training or competing.

Besides using a refractometer, athletes can assess their own hydration status by simply using urine color and body-weight markers. Using both concurrently is recommended to minimize any limitations that one individual marker may present. Ideally, testing the first urine of the morning for color and specific gravity and monitoring body weight should provide enough information to detect any changes in water balance. It is of utmost importance that the first void of the day be used for analysis and interpretation because it will reflect hydration status better than later in the day, when there are various items that will manipulate the measurement.

Using a urine color chart to assess hydration status has grown in popularity, and it is important to understand the basis for this tool. The color of urine is determined primarily by the amount of urochrome, which is a breakdown product of hemoglobin. When a large amount of urine is excreted, the urine is dilute and the substances in the urine are excreted in large amounts. This gives the urine a pale color. When a small amount of urine is excreted, the urine is more concentrated and the solutes are excreted in smaller amounts. This gives the urine a darker color. The urine color chart includes a scale of eight colors that show a linear relationship between the color of urine and the specific gravity and osmolality of urine. These colors are described in table 2.6 on page 39. When using this assessment tool, remember that certain dietary compounds can affect the color of urine, including B-complex vitamins, carotene, betacyanins, and some artificial food colors. Athletes should pay particular attention to these factors if they frequently use urine color to determine hydration status.

Body weight can also be used as a somewhat effective hydration status tool, but it should be noted that an athlete's training nutrition, specifically carbohydrate intake, can affect glycogen storage. Glycogen stores more water, and thus body weight can be artificially altered simply based on carbohydrate intake and training status. For well-hydrated people who are in energy balance, body-weight fluctuations should be plus or minus 1 percent when measured in the morning after urinating. However, it is best to confirm this with the color of the urine since body weight can be affected by things other than fluid loss or gain.

Closely monitoring body weight before and after training also allows athletes to calculate their sweat rate, which can be used to create fluid replacement strategies. See page 39 for instructions on how to calculate sweat rate.

Hydration and Performance

Maintaining fluid and electrolyte balance is crucial for athletes because a fluid loss of 2 percent of body weight has been shown to reduce exercise performance (figure 5.1). However, there is not total agreement on the level of body-weight loss before performance is reduced. In one particular study of Ironman triathletes, a 3 percent reduction in body mass during competition showed that thermoregulation was maintained, and body core temperature did not rise enough to lead to heat stroke, which may indicate that some athletes may be better regulators of heat and require different fluid strategies. Common sense has proved this to be true, and most athletes and coaches can attest that certain times of the year require differences in hydration techniques for certain athletes. In another study looking at anaerobic power using Wingate testing, a 2.9 percent body-weight loss decreased the body's ability to generate upper- and lower-body power. This is of utmost importance for strength and power athletes throughout the training year because being in a dehydrated state, also known as **hypohydration,** before training sessions can lead to a reduction in work, which can carry over to impaired performance during competition.

hypohydration – An insufficient amount of water.

It is generally believed that exercise that results in dehydration can also have debilitating effects on mental performance, including concentration, mood state, and reaction time. This is of particular concern to athletes who are required to complete both simple and complex tasks in their sports. As is usually the case, there is research to both prove and dispute this fact, but because mental performance and its associated

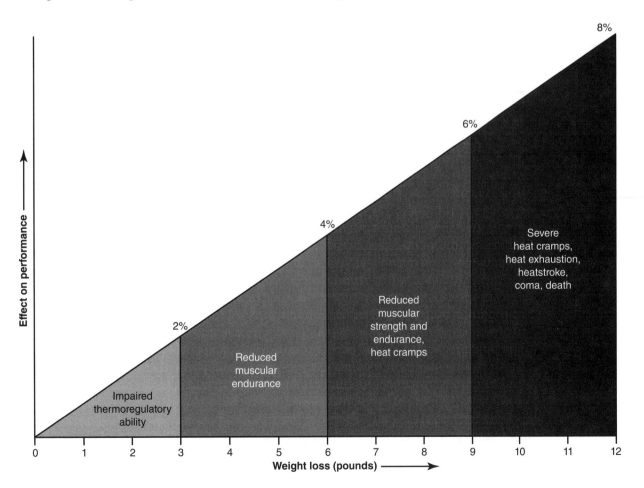

Figure 5.1 Effects of dehydration on physical performance, by body weight lost, on a 150-pound (68 kg) athlete.

Managing Hydration and a High Sweat Rate

A world-class taekwondo athlete experienced symptoms of blurred vision only on competition days. The athlete was observed during training, and it was noted that he was sweating significantly. His hydration status was monitored over several days, revealing that the athlete walked around in a chronic state of dehydration that was equivalent to approximately 4 percent of his body mass. Assessment of sweat rate, by weighing the athlete before and after training in dry clothing, revealed that he was losing the equivalent of 2.5 liters of fluid per hour during even a moderate training session with very intermittent bouts of sparring. It was thought that a full 10-hour day of competition may be dehydrating the athlete to a point that the blurred vision was due to significant dehydration.

The athlete did not have a plan for taking in fluids for rehydration on a day-to-day basis or for competition because it was not commonplace in his sport. A primary concern about full rehydration was the increase in body mass that this would represent for the athlete when weighed on the scale; however, once the athlete was educated on dehydration, its effects, and the fact that the change in weight was only a result of water in the body, he could accept the higher body weight. In addition, the athlete developed a timing system for taking in fluid to replace what was lost in training while also learning to sip on fluid during training.

Once the athlete had learned to take in fluid, an additional intervention was used to reduce the athlete's sweat rate. An ice vest that could easily be repeatedly cooled and worn underneath the ghee (uniform) was used before and after each round of the tournament. This procedure reduced the sweat rate by .8 liters per hour and provided an additional psychological benefit to the athlete during competition.

factors have been shown to decline with dehydration, athletes and coaches should pay particular attention to hydration status. The sensation of thirst can also influence behavior and cognitive performance. Many research studies have discovered that in dehydrated states ranging from 1 to 5 percent, people can experience increased fatigue, reduced speed and accuracy when doing complicated tasks, impaired short-term memory and attention, and increased reaction time. This obviously has potential performance-reducing implications for all athletes regardless of the sport. Because cognitive function drives movement patterns and decision making relating to tactical and technical implementation in sport, it is important for all athletes to remain as hydrated as possible during competition and quality training sessions where improving performance is the main objective. In addition, athletes should mimic competition-day hydration strategies during training sessions.

Preexercise Hydration

To achieve the physical and mental goals of a training session, athletes must begin exercise euhydrated and with normal electrolyte levels. Good hydration practices during the day focus on the consumption of water and foods containing water, such as fruits and vegetables. If at least 8 hours have passed since the last training session and sufficient fluids have been consumed with meals, the athlete should be close to an euhydrated state. However, if an athlete had a particularly challenging training session in the last 24 hours that resulted in a significant amount of fluid lost, a more aggressive preexercise hydration protocol should be implemented.

Immediately before exercise, it is recommended that athletes consume .07 to .10 ounces of fluid per pound (4.7 to 6.6 ml/kg) of body weight at least 4 hours beforehand.

More fluid should be consumed—approximately .04 to .10 ounces per pound (2.7 to 6.6 ml/kg) of body weight—2 hours before if an athlete has not urinated or the urine is dark in color. For example, a 170-pound (77 kg) athlete would drink 11.9 to 17 ounces (360 to 510 ml) of fluid 4 hours before training and an additional 6.8 to 17 ounces (210 to 510 ml) of fluid 2 hours beforehand.

It is important for athletes to include higher-sodium foods to stimulate thirst and retain fluids. Consuming sodium in a sports drink is an easy method of obtaining the necessary fluid, carbohydrate, and sodium needed before a training session or competition.

A common practice before an event is for athletes to attempt to hyperhydrate with water alone, which can act as a diuretic. This is not advised because it will increase the risk of urination during the competition and could dilute the sodium levels in the body, thus increasing the risk of hyponatremia. To promote a euhydrated state before training or competition, fluid palatability is of utmost importance. A good recommendation is a beverage that is lightly sweetened, contains sodium, and is a cool temperature.

Timeline

Hydration Timeline
- **4 hours before exercise:** .07 to .10 oz/lb (4.7 to 6.6 ml/kg) of body weight
- **2 hours before exercise:** .04 to .10 oz/lb (2.7 to 6.6 ml/kg) of body weight
- **During exercise:** 3 to 8 oz (90 to 240 ml) every 15 to 20 minutes
- **After exercise:** 24 oz/lb (1.6 L/kg) of body weight lost

Hydration During Exercise

The goal of drinking during exercise is to prevent excessive dehydration, which has a negative impact on performance, and excessive changes in electrolyte balance, which could lead to hyponatremia. Although fluid replacement strategies are highly individualized, consuming between 3 and 8 ounces (90 and 240 ml) of a carbohydrate–

Athletes in combative or contact sports often find it difficult to have any fluid in the stomach during competition.

electrolyte fluid every 15 to 20 minutes will assist in hydration status and promote better performance in exercise longer than 60 minutes. Whenever possible, athletes should maintain the frequency of these fluid intervals to allow the body to receive a consistent amount of hydration. It is also better to take larger gulps than small sips as this will speed the time that the fluid empties from the stomach, which can help reduce gastrointestinal distress. Depending on sweat rate and environment, an athlete may need more or less fluids per hour.

Depending on the sport, however, consuming 3 to 8 ounces (90 to 240 ml) every 15 to 20 minutes may not be realistic or viable. Specifically, athletes who compete in sports that do not have frequent breaks; combative sports such as wrestling, taekwondo, and boxing; or sports that vibrate the GI system such as running or cross-country skiing would find it extremely difficult to drink much fluid. In these cases, it is important that the athlete adhere closely to the precompetition fluid recommendations in order to enter training and competition in a well-hydrated state. These athletes may not drink much during, but they can start training or competition with a relatively full tank. This has been proven in many environmental conditions in both males and females with various exercise modes, durations, and intensities and is fairly easy to do with some preplanning work from the athlete and coach.

Consuming carbohydrate during exercise maintains blood glucose levels and reduces fatigue. The Institute of Medicine recommends a sports drink containing 460 to 1,150 mg of sodium per liter and 78 to 195 mg of potassium per liter. This combination can also be consumed from energy bars and gels and other foods depending on a person's needs and preferences.

However, if you are in a training cycle in which you are actively trying to lose weight, consuming a sports drink during practice will slow your progress. Instead, choose water with added electrolytes as your main hydration beverage. The only time to consider an exception would be when training 3 or more hours during hot and humid conditions, especially if you are a heavy sweater.

Postexercise Hydration

After exercise, the goal is to fully replenish any fluid and electrolyte deficit experienced from the training session in order to return to normal before the next workout or competition. Consuming 150 percent of weight loss is required to achieve normal hydration within 6 hours after exercise. Therefore, practically speaking, it is recommended that 24 ounces (720 ml) of fluids be consumed for every pound (.45 kg) of body weight an athlete loses after training. Plain water is not an effective rehydrator, and it should only be included in the postworkout plan when it is combined with higher-sodium foods. Over a period of 8 to 24 hours, water losses can be fully replaced to establish normal total body water, within .2 to .5 percent of starting weight if adequate fluid and electrolytes are consumed.

Depending on the amount of time an athlete has before the next exercise session, water and sodium-rich foods and beverages after competition or a training session should suffice. Sodium is one of the key nutrients to consume in the postexercise period to return to a euhydrated state because it will help retain fluids consumed and stimulate thirst. Although sweat sodium losses differ among athletes, which makes individual sodium prescription difficult during this period, a little extra salt added to meals or snacks may be particularly useful for those with high sweat sodium losses. Other than having sweat sodium concentration tested in a laboratory setting, a quick visual test to determine if an athlete loses a high amount of sodium in sweat is to look for any white residue (salt) on the face, clothing, or body during or after a workout. If white residue is visible, it may be indicative of a high sweat sodium concentration.

Adapting the Hydration Timeline

The hydration guidelines should be adapted to suit the needs of each individual athlete, based on the athlete's sweat rate, type of sport, and ability to tolerate fluid during exercise. Here is an example of how the hydration timeline could be adapted for a male recreational marathon runner who cannot tolerate much fluid while running and does not normally consume much water before or during training runs. This runner lives in hot and humid conditions and has a high sweat rate with a high sweat sodium concentration, which makes the hydration and electrolyte plan even more important. If this athlete is going for a long run of 2 hours, the overall fluid amounts before and during the run may need to be decreased. A sports drink can be used in place of water to help maintain sodium levels during exercise. After exercise, this athlete should follow the rehydration recommendations to replace fluid lost.

4 hours before exercise: .04 to .10 oz of sports drink per lb (2.7 to 6.6 ml/kg) of body weight

2 hours before exercise: .04 to .07 oz of sports drink per lb (2.7 to 4.7 ml/kg) of body weight

During exercise: Sips of water or sports drink whenever possible

30 to 60 minutes after exercise: 24 oz of fluid for every lb (1.6 L for every kg) of body weight lost

Hydration Issues

Certain conditions relating to hydration and athletes are important to understand. These include hyponatremia, exercise-associated muscle cramps, and planned dehydration strategies for certain groups of athletes, all of which can have a negative effect on performance and health if not accounted for in the hydration plan.

Hyponatremia

Exercise-associated hyponatremia, a low concentration of sodium in the blood, is very common in many athletes and can be deadly. Although the exact cause is not known, contributing factors include overdrinking hypotonic fluids, an excessive loss of sodium through sweat, and heavy sweating while drinking low-sodium fluids. In general, hyponatremia that happens in events lasting less than 4 hours can usually be caused by simply overdrinking, or **hyperhydration,** before and during competition. This is a somewhat interesting topic because athletes are normally told to hydrate beforehand and during exercise and by no means is this incorrect. The point is that some athletes overconsume fluids to try to hyperhydrate, and when water is the only beverage used for this, it typically leads to a diluted sodium content and thus hyponatremia.

hyperhydration – An excess amount of water.

Female athletes may be at higher risk of developing hyponatremia in longer endurance events, possibly for a number of psychosocial and biological reasons such as different hormonal responses; in addition, fluid intake recommendations for women have been often based on sweat loss data from men. These numbers would obviously be too high for women based on body size differences, and this itself may be a main reason for a higher incidence of hyponatremia. Because of these size differences, it is very important that female athletes individualize their fluid and electrolyte intake based on their bodies and sweat rate and not on male counterparts.

There is no exact recommendation regarding electrolyte intake before exercise, although many athletes consume salty foods and beverages beforehand to reduce the risk of hyponatremia. For heavy sweaters or athletes training and competing in a hot and humid environment, increasing the amount of daily salt eaten in foods may be necessary, in addition to consuming more salt before, during, and after training. Some athletes use electrolyte supplements to achieve this, and as long as they are consumed with enough fluid, this is another option for athletes at high risk of developing hyponatremia.

Exercise-Associated Muscle Cramps (EAMCs)

It is common for athletes to experience muscle cramps as a result of exercising. Although usually not life threatening, these cramping incidents can debilitate an athlete for some time and lead to decreased performance. EAMCs happen frequently in endurance sports such as triathlon, where up to 67 percent of athletes have been affected, while 18 to 70 percent of marathoners and endurance cyclists have been affected. Even in team sports, such as American football, there is a relatively high incidence rate ranging from 30 to 53 percent. Unfortunately, the causes of cramping have not been well defined.

Prevention is the obvious goal for all athletes and coaches. The most common proposed causes of EAMCs relate to dehydration, environmental stress (heat and humidity), and low sodium concentrations in the body. The main electrolytes that can delay the onset of EAMCs include sodium, chloride, potassium, magnesium, and calcium. These are the predominant electrolytes found in sweat and therefore should be the main focal points for athletes. Individual variability should be considered when devising a proper fluid and electrolyte plan because some athletes have a higher incidence of cramping when consuming carbohydrate and electrolytes rather than just water. It is important to note an athlete's sport, position if applicable, training environments, and training status. For example, a runner who is training outdoors during the wintertime in the mountains of Colorado may not need as much fluid as if the run were taking place indoors on a treadmill. If a boxer normally trains in a hotter environment to promote sweat loss, hydration and electrolyte needs would be, theoretically, increased, although in specific instances during weight cutting, these practices may not be followed well. What is important is understanding the intricacies of the sport's requirements, fluid needs, body-weight goals, and opportunities to implement a hydration and electrolyte plan.

Planned Dehydration

A hydration and electrolyte plan can become complex at times for certain athletes. Take an ultraendurance runner as an example. Opportunities to hydrate may be minimal because of the duration of training, and the ability to carry enough fluid is reduced because of the sport (wanting to be as light as possible to improve economy and speed). As a result, ultra-endurance runners may attempt to train their bodies to perform in a semi-dehydrated state, and therefore, their bodies would adapt. It is virtually impossible for most ultraendurance athletes to prevent dehydration due to fluid losses through sweat. This further supports these athletes' attempts to teach their bodies the "less is more" principle of hydration because of their sport's limitations and their bodies' physiological responses to training. During endurance competitions, it becomes more important to attempt to delay dehydration than to prevent it.

For weight-classified athletes such as wrestlers, hydration practices are very unique. For these athletes, fluid is commonly manipulated to make a specified weight, but the key traits that make a wrestler successful (strength, power, and anaerobic endurance) can be easily compromised with even two percent dehydration. In addition, techniques used in the sport (e.g., gut-wrench technique) frequently involve pressure on the stomach and being thrown during competition, which could potentially result in vomiting if the stomach contains too much food or fluid, so consuming a lot of fluid just before competition is usually impractical.

At the high school and collegiate levels, wrestling competitions start 30 minutes to 2 hours after weighing in. As a result, there is very little time to recover fluids lost through dehydration to make weight, and it is not recommended that athletes not lose any more than 2 to 3 percent of body weight through dehydration (assuming they are in a fully euhydrated state to begin). The time frame for rehydration is short, and for most athletes the maximum rate at which fluid empties from the stomach is on average 16 to 20 ounces (480 to 600 ml) every 15 minutes. The ability of the stomach to empty fluid is highly dependent on the athlete's having previously trained the gut to do so; otherwise the rate of emptying is slower since the body is unaccustomed to it. This emphasizes the need for weight-classified athletes to consistently follow good hydration practices. The other factor that must be considered is how well an athlete can consume fluid in relation to competition readiness. Many athletes are nervous or have some form of anxiety going into major competitions; as a result it may be best for the athlete to compete at a weight where dehydration is not necessary.

At national and international levels, there is typically at least 18 hours between weigh-in and competition. These athletes could potentially lose up to 5 percent of body mass (assuming a fully euhydrated state to begin) through dehydration to make their designated weight class; however, this is variable by athlete and dependent on sweat rate, ability to rehydrate, and tolerance to heat exposure for dehydration. Research has shown that dehydration beyond 5 percent of body mass will affect muscular performance, and thus it is not recommended. The "In Practice" section shows rehydration timelines to use after a weight cut. For a detailed example of a precompetition weight strategy for a wrestler, see chapter 10.

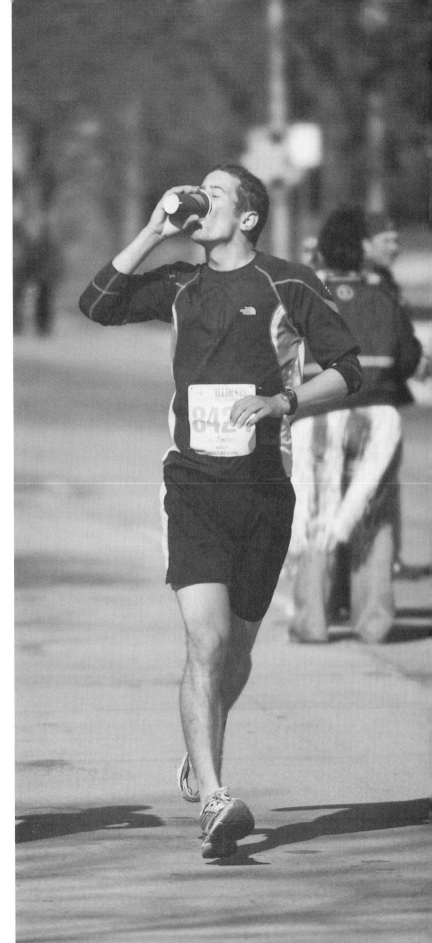

Whenever possible, athletes should drink at frequent intervals during exercise and competition to maintain hydration.

Hydration Timeline for a Combative Sport

Most sports that are combative in nature compete in rounds that begin at approximately 9:00 a.m. and end later in the evening. Athletes frequently must make weight and do so through some form of dehydration. Although wrestlers are usually leery of consuming food and fluids during competition, fluids can replenish fuel stores and help athletes recover from making weight. Fluid intake is trainable, and the recovery timeline should be dependent on the amount of time between the weigh-in and competition.

RECOVERY PLAN: EIGHTEEN HOURS BETWEEN WEIGH-IN AND COMPETITION

Here is a sample recovery pattern timeline for an athlete with 18 hours between weigh-in and competition. This is most common for wrestling at the national and international levels and tae-kwondo athletes at all levels.

These are minimums for an athlete who dehydrated by 5 percent of body mass and weighed in at 108 pounds (49 kg).

First priority: Replace lost fluids and electrolytes.

Second priority: Recover carbohydrates.

First 2.5 hours after weigh-in:

Immediately after: 12 oz (360 ml) carbohydrate–electrolyte beverage + water to taste

30 minutes after: 12 oz (360 ml) carbohydrate–electrolyte beverage + water to taste

Food–Nibble: pretzels, crackers, white bread, salty foods, and so on; avoid high fat and too much protein

60 minutes after: 12 oz (360 ml) carbohydrate–electrolyte beverage + water to taste

Food–Nibble: same

90 minutes after: 12 oz (360 ml) carbohydrate–electrolyte beverage + water to taste

Food–Nibble: same

120 minutes after: 6 oz (180 ml) carbohydrate–electrolyte beverage + water to taste

Food–Nibble: same

150 minutes after: 6 oz (180 ml) carbohydrate–electrolyte beverage + water to taste

Food–Nibble: same

Continue sipping fluids all evening to ensure rehydration is complete!

Meal

- Let the recovery food settle, and enjoy your meal.
- Ensure your meal is low glycemic and contains lean protein and starchy carbohydrates.
- Stay away from vegetables that are high in fiber content.
- Stick to fluids with electrolytes (e.g., juice, milk, Gatorade) and water to taste and other noncarbonated beverages.

Before Bed

- Have a glass of milk or chocolate milk.

Competition Day

- Breakfast should be familiar.
- Consume at least two glasses of water upon wakening.
- Consume at least 250 calories every 3 hours.
- Use sipping and nibbling technique to keep food and fluids down and comfortable.
- Consume larger amounts in the time periods between rounds that are further apart so that food has adequate time to digest.
- Remember: Eat low-residue foods, and rotate water and carbohydrate–electrolyte beverages.

RECOVERY PLAN: TWO HOURS BETWEEN WEIGH-IN AND COMPETITION

Here is a sample recovery pattern timeline for an athlete with 2 hours or less between weigh-in and competition. This is most common for wrestling at the high school and collegiate levels, judo, and boxing.

These are minimums for an athlete who dehydrated by 3 percent of body mass and weighed in at 108 pounds (49 kg).

First priority: Replace lost fluids and electrolytes.

Second priority: Recover carbohydrates.

First 2 hours after weigh-in:

Immediately after: 12 oz (360 ml) carbohydrate–electrolyte beverage + water to taste

30 minutes after: 12 oz (360 ml) carbohydrate–electrolyte beverage + water to taste

Food–Nibble: pretzels, crackers, white bread, salty foods, and so on; avoid high fat and too much protein.

60 to 120 minutes after: 12 oz (360 ml) carbohydrate–electrolyte beverage + water to taste

Food–Nibble: same

Continue nibbling on food that is low in residue and has a low to moderate glycemic response as can be tolerated. Consume larger amounts in the time periods between rounds that are further apart so that food has adequate time to digest.

If heat exposure is used for dehydration, the athlete must be conditioned to tolerate heat. Tolerance to the heat is highly dependent on using a proper heat acclimation process and on the level of body fat the athlete maintains. Acclimation to the heat (at least 14 days with at least 2 days in between to assist with the fever) is necessary so the body becomes accustomed to this additional demand being placed on it. Athletes who have high levels of body fat cannot easily dissipate heat and will have a decreased ability to make weight using heat exposure. The addition of cooling techniques (e.g., cool towels, hand immersion in cool water) to help facilitate recovery from the use of a sauna or other techniques used for dehydration will also become important.

During training and competition, most athletes cannot handle much food or fluid in the stomach. As a result, hydration for the most part must be done before training and resume immediately after it ceases. It is beneficial to teach the body to adapt to performing in a state of dehydration during training because, in competition, athletes may have several bouts close together and do not have time to process any substantial amount of fluid. A sipping (or gulping) protocol should be developed for in-competition use.

Conclusion

Fluid and electrolyte consumption during training and competition should be customized to the athlete, the sport, and its requirements. Clear performance declines are seen with voluntary or forced dehydration in all types of athletes, from endurance to power and strength. Athletes should implement proper hydration techniques throughout training in an effort to improve performance in competition along with maintaining adequate fluid levels during competition itself.

Macronutrient Timing Strategies

An athlete's diet should be balanced in its macronutrient distribution to meet the essential vitamins and minerals as well as minimize illness, injury, and disease. The macronutrients should also be distributed to support the energy demands of training. The goal of this chapter is to explain how the macronutrients can be utilized under the concept of nutrient timing to achieve an athlete's goals for performance nutrition. This primarily centers around what an athlete should eat before, during, and after training as well as in between training sessions. In addition, this chapter demonstrates how proper timing of the macronutrients can build an athlete's energy systems, thus improving the physical capacity to do work.

The use of macronutrients to manipulate a nutrition plan must meet what is commonly known as the recommended dietary allowances (RDAs). The RDA is the amount of a nutrient that is necessary for most people to sustain life. This is also commonly used in conjunction with the dietary reference intakes (DRIs). The DRIs are a set of nutrient-based values that can be used to evaluate how nutritious a diet is. They evaluate the minimal amount needed, the average requirement, and what the upper intake level can be without compromising the body and health. For an athlete, a key component of using the RDAs and DRIs is how they are distributed in the diet—in other words, the percentage of calories coming from protein, carbohydrate, and fat. The DRIs express this distribution as the acceptable macronutrient distribution range (AMDR). Acceptable macronutrient distribution ranges (as a percentage of calories) are as follows: protein, 10 to 35 percent; fat, 20 to 35 percent; and carbohydrate, 45 to 65 percent. An athlete's nutrient timing system should be designed to strategically utilize the distribution of the macronutrients to meet performance and training goals while simultaneously meeting the RDAs to support health.

This chapter provides strategies that are intended for both short- and long-term manipulation of the macronutrients. Short-term strategies are designed for periods of three to five days and are intended to create a very specific training adaptation. Long-term strategies are designed to optimize an athlete's health and support training goals. Although short-term strategies may not always fall within the AMDR, this has not been shown to have any consequence on health or performance. Long-term strategies incorporate the AMDR to ensure that, first and foremost, health is maintained; second, they show how to manipulate the timing of the macronutrients to optimize their use throughout the training day.

Nutrient Strategies

This chapter is divided by the macronutrients, and recommendations are based on the intensity of training and the specific goals athletes have for their sports. The key to strategically utilizing the macronutrients is to gain an understanding of what an athlete needs based on the intensity, duration, and technical aspects of the sport. Athletes from all types of sports can recognize the importance of maintaining a high ratio of muscle to fat mass for performance advantages, and thus using a timing strategy to optimize food intake is a key aspect of an athlete's periodization.

Endurance sports are greater than 3 minutes in continuous duration and rely heavily on the aerobic energy system. They include rowing, triathlon, distance running, ultraendurance events, cross-country skiing, and biathlon. These types of sports require athletes to maintain a relatively low level of body fat, as this can assist with aerobic economy to supply the power required for covering long distances.

Technical sports such as shooting, archery, and equestrian all require long days of training and competition. Although the intensity of training is not high, strength, muscular endurance, and mental stamina are required for success. Competitions are often held outdoors in warm environments, and thus athletes prefer to be lean and slim. In a sport such as equestrian, athletes are also frequently judged by their appearance before they even begin to compete.

Sports that are acrobatic in nature such as gymnastics and synchronized swimming require large volumes of technical training, along with training for muscular strength and power that will allow athletes to explode and recover quickly for repeated bouts in a routine. In combative sports, athletes are classified by weight, and one of the greatest focuses is managing weight while still being able to sustain high-intensity training bouts that require explosive strength. Appetite control is critical because acrobatic sports require an unusually small body size that is lean, and combative sports frequently require athletes to train at the lowest body weight that can be sustained for the athlete's height.

In strength and power events such as sprinting, throwing, weightlifting, and bobsledding, athletes consistently look to optimize the amount of force they can produce per pound of muscle mass. Training volume is rarely high but is very intense. It is also not uncommon for athletes to desire increases in size through gains in muscle mass.

In team sports, such as soccer, baseball, basketball, and football, athletes must develop a large anaerobic capacity as well as strength and power endurance. These athletes must be able to repeatedly sprint with very little recovery. They are also required to carry their body weight in many different directions; thus, economy of movement is a key component to success. This is highly facilitated through maintaining a body composition that does not have excess fat mass and will not increase the energy cost of running and changing direction.

All of these sports require optimal recovery and muscle maintenance; however, each allows for very different levels of energy intake. The optimal composition of athletes' diets will depend highly on the sport they are engaged in, their ability to derive energy from carbohydrate and fat stores, the type of training they need to undertake, and whether body composition or weight is a factor that needs to be manipulated. This chapter discusses each macronutrient and then shows how to systematically determine macronutrient intake before, during, and after training. Throughout the chapter, you will see sample nutrition timelines for three athletes, showing recommendations for training and competition. These timelines show how the principles in this chapter can be tailored to the unique needs of every athlete.

Pretraining Nutrient Strategies

The amount of carbohydrate, protein, and fat consumed has a substantial impact on how quickly the fuel is delivered and utilized by the body. This is extremely important for athletes who implement feeding strategies to improve performance in training and competition. It also plays a significant role in the ability to gain muscle mass and lose body fat. The greatest benefits of the macronutrients are met when considering the training goals.

Carbohydrate Intake Before Training and Competition

Eating before a training session is very specific to the athlete and sport, but the underlying goal is that athletes have enough energy to sustain their physical efforts during the session. Carbohydrates provide this energy, and athletes should enter training sessions as well fueled with carbohydrate as possible. However, because of differences in body composition and intensity of the sport as well as individual sensitivity of the digestive system, one strategy may be good for one athlete yet have a negative impact on another athlete.

Carbohydrate consumption before, during, and after training should be based on the goals of the training session. When it is important to maintain a high intensity and strong work capacity throughout the session, carbohydrate ingestion before and during can be beneficial, and it is highly important to ensure that this fuel is readily available to the body. However, if a training session is meant to promote a metabolic and physiological adaptation, such as improving fat utilization during rest and exercise, the ingestion of carbohydrate would actually hinder this process. Thus, the timing of carbohydrate ingestion must consider the training goal. Most athletes find that a more balanced feeding 1 to 2 hours before training, consisting of carbohydrate with a little protein and fat, sits better in their system and controls their blood sugar and energy levels. Overall, athletes may respond better to liquid sources of carbohydrate such as sports drinks than to solid foods. Additionally, lower-fiber foods may be beneficial to some athletes who have sensitive digestive systems.

The type of carbohydrate consumed, along with any protein and fat, should produce a low glycemic response that does not raise blood glucose and then cause rebound hypoglycemia. In sports where prolonged high-intensity training sessions predominate, sufficient carbohydrate must be consumed in the hour before to ensure that glycogen stores are adequate. This typically requires an average intake of 1 to 1.5 grams of carbohydrate per kilogram of body weight (.5 to .7 grams per pound) in the hour before and then a continuous dribble of carbohydrate up until the start. The range, however, may be as low as .5 g/kg of body weight in an aesthetic sport such as synchronized swimming where weight control is crucial and as high as 3 g/kg of body weight in a larger athlete who participates in a sport such as football and must maintain and may even be looking to increase body mass.

Protein Intake Before Training and Competition

Since what we know about protein is in relation to creating a training response, a good starting point for determining an athlete's protein intake is to organize the intake around training and its goals. Once protein intake is situated to support training, then the remainder can be strategically placed to meet goals for body composition, weight management, and essential requirements for daily needs.

The timing of protein intake is known to facilitate muscle synthesis, repair, and maintenance; enhance recovery from training through improving muscle glycogen stores; enhance sleep quality; and maintain stable blood glucose levels. Fast proteins (whey or amino acids), slow proteins (casein), or a combination of both can be ingested through foods or supplements to meet the timeline requirements for achieving training goals. Protein can also be used to control appetite and improve the glycemic response of a food. The timing, type, and functionality of a food must be brought together to achieve the training response.

Because protein can contribute to muscle synthesis and prevent muscle breakdown during training, the timing of protein intake before training is dependent on whether or not an athlete is looking to stimulate increases in muscle synthesis or just maintain what is already present. The intake of protein needed to stimulate muscle synthesis can range from 6 to 20 grams; in order for athletes to maintain or increase muscle mass, large amounts of protein are not necessary.

Gaining body weight in the form of muscle is dependent on the caloric density of foods consumed around training, especially resistance training. The relationship to resistance training is a key component of the equation. If a coach just gives an athlete protein and extra calories, there is a very slim chance that the athlete would increase muscle mass; most likely, he would increase his fat mass. However, when increased caloric intake is centered around resistance training, research has shown that muscle growth is not only stimulated but also highly accentuated. This response has been seen with a wide range of protein intakes. Anywhere from 6 to 20 grams of protein along with a serving of carbohydrate 30 minutes before resistance training has been shown to increase muscle synthesis. This may be even further enhanced through the consumption of an additional bolus of protein, carbohydrate, and fat within the 2-hour period after training. This pattern must be sustained to ensure that weight gain occurs over time.

Muscle synthesis in response to training may be best facilitated through dairy products that contain both whey (fast) and casein (slow) proteins, which will provide protein during the training bout and after training to sustain muscle repair and synthesis. It is not feasible for all athletes to consume dairy products because of lactose intolerance. Foods such as lactose-free meal-replacement shakes, meats, fish, soy, and nuts mixed with other foods items can also supply the protein necessary to achieve this goal. Although natural foods are always best, some athletes may prefer to use supplements (protein powders) to facilitate this process. Supplementation to meet the demands of increased muscle protein synthesis can be done by providing a whey protein plus carbohydrate bolus before training and then a casein-based protein plus carbohydrate and fat bolus after the training session.

Athletes looking to sustain the muscle mass they already have and who may also want to convert fat mass to muscle mass through a resistance training program do not need such caloric density. A low-fat protein source in the 30 minutes before resistance training, with no more than 13 grams of protein, is enough to meet this training goal. This may be accomplished through low-fat dairy products, lean meats, or protein powders. The other key aspect is the caloric density athletes have in their diet on the whole. The body will continue to gain mass (fat or muscle) when energy intake exceeds expenditure; thus, it is equally important that athletes monitor the remainder of the food intake and ensure that energy balance is maintained.

For athletes who need to sustain muscle mass and must watch body weight closely, food intake before resistance training is not needed. Free-form essential amino acids (leucine, isoleucine, valine), which do not provide a high caloric density, could be consumed to minimize muscle breakdown, especially when in a period of caloric restriction.

Protein intake before competition is highly dependent on individual digestion patterns and whether or not protein might inhibit the absorption of carbohydrate necessary for sustaining energy. High-intensity endurance and team sports typically require that athletes minimize protein intake in the 2 hours before competition for this very reason. Conversely, athletes in sports such as equestrian and shooting that do not require high levels of carbohydrate to sustain energy levels may utilize protein to minimize hunger and produce a low glycemic response while still allowing the athlete to eat in the lead-up to and throughout the competition. To determine whether or not protein is appropriate for an athlete, coaches must consider the energy systems used, the potential for energy depletion to occur, and how it makes the athlete feel. Typically, sports with higher energy demands will minimize protein intake, while those with minimal energy expenditure will allow for higher levels of protein intake.

Fat Intake Before Training and Competition

Fat loading, or following a high-fat diet for days or weeks leading up to a competition, has been widely studied with varying results. Some research indicates that consuming more fat in the diet increases fat availability for exercise, but the performance improvements have been argued, and if seen, they are small and at lower exercise intensities. Following a high-fat diet (>60 to 65 percent of total energy intake) for up to 28 days has been shown to increase fat oxidation and decrease the rate of muscle glycogen use, but only during submaximal exercise. What is certain is that if athletes increase fat in the diet in the hope of improving performance during competition, adaptations can be achieved in as little as five days. This brief exposure to this type of nutrition program is preferred over a longer lasting adaptation period, which may sacrifice an athlete's ability to maintain high-intensity training leading up to competition and would thus compromise performance.

Several types of athletes may consider a high-fat diet before competition or as a training intervention. Athletes who want to improve the body's ability to preserve muscle glycogen stores during prolonged competitions and the aerobic energy system's ability to utilize fat as a fuel source may attempt a high-fat diet for a period of approximately five days. This strategy should help prevent fatigue and improve recovery for those athletes competing in multiple events throughout the day. This could apply to endurance athletes who require a significant contribution from the aerobic energy system during competition; in the case of sprint and middle-distance swimmers, the goal may be to increase the aerobic energy system to improve the body's ability to utilize fat as a fuel source and reduce the reliance on muscle glycogen stores. In both scenarios, athletes can benefit by minimizing the buildup of lactate, preserving glycogen stores, and improving aerobic metabolism.

It is important that athletes reduce the amount of fat in their normal nutrition plans in the hours to days (depending on the athlete and whether it is a weight-class sport) leading up to competition in order to properly replenish glycogen stores. This strategy ensures full regeneration of muscle glycogen stores by allowing for more carbohydrate intake. Athletes who perform glycogen-depleting sports will benefit from this strategy. This includes team sports such as soccer, basketball, and ice hockey as well as endurance sports and technical strength and power sports such as tennis and volleyball. Dietary fat intake should be minimal to normal, with special attention given to promoting more omega-3 fats to reduce inflammation and medium-chain triglycerides to improve intramuscular triglyceride stores; saturated and trans fats that can inhibit gastric emptying and increase oxidative stress should be minimized.

Nutrient Strategies During Training

Strategies of nutrient timing during training are typically done to increase energy capacity (i.e., the amount of work an athlete can perform), minimize fatigue, or simulate a competition-like situation. These strategies are generally geared toward teaching the body to produce a greater amount of power with a desired energy source (e.g., fat or carbohydrate), and as a result work capacity increases. Increased energy supply to minimize fatigue helps reduce muscle damage and decrease the amount of time a muscle spends in a catabolic state (muscle breakdown) and the amount of time necessary to recover from a hard training bout. In the third scenario, athletes practice consuming an increased level of nutrient intake to ensure they are comfortable with the strategies that will help sustain performance during competition.

Carbohydrate Intake During Training and Competition

As mentioned previously, carbohydrate provides the body with a significant amount of energy during moderate- to high-intensity exercise. Depending on the sport and

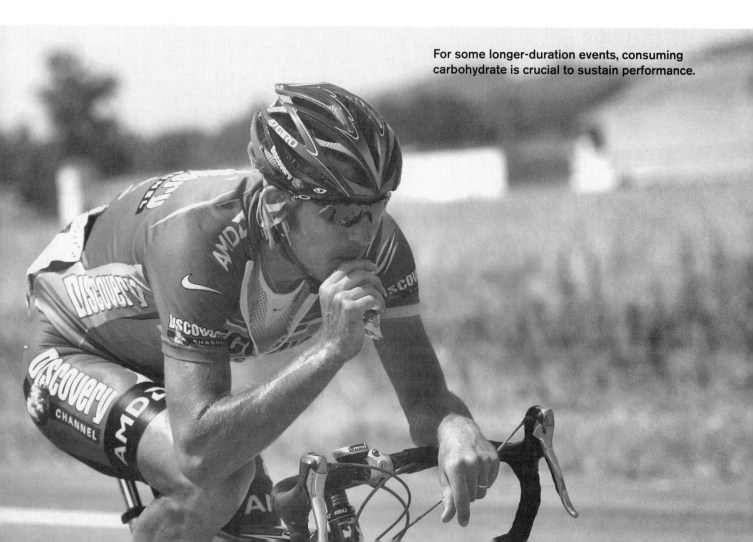

For some longer-duration events, consuming carbohydrate is crucial to sustain performance.

its associated breaks, it may be very important to consume carbohydrate during training and competition in order to sustain the quality of work being performed. For most sports, carbohydrate sources that provide a steady supply of carbohydrate without spike and crash patterns in blood glucose benefit the athletes more as this will sustain fuel to the working muscles. Refer to chapter 4 for specific timing and quantity of carbohydrate consumption, but in general, sources such as sports drinks, energy gels, bars, and chews are popular among athletes. Some athletes also consume preformulated drinks and shakes to deliver more of a balance of carbohydrate, protein, and fat. Most important is the frequency of carbohydrate feeding as it relates to the duration of training or the competition bout and the amount needed in order to maintain stable blood glucose levels as much as possible throughout the training session or competition.

The intake of carbohydrate during training and competition is highly dependent on the needs of each athlete. Some athletes require a substantially larger amount of carbohydrate than do others depending on how well the body is able to utilize fat as a fuel source and the amount of time spent competing. This can vary widely by sport depending on position played or the duration of the competition. Think of an athlete competing in a marathon in comparison to the 5,000 meters on the track, or in the case of a team sport, a baseball pitcher pitching for multiple innings while another player bats in only a few innings and doesn't even have to run for first base.

Regardless of the sport, athletes need to consume a form of carbohydrate that can easily empty from the stomach and does not cause gastrointestinal distress. Gastrointestinal distress typically occurs as a result of consuming carbohydrate in too high of a concentration or too much fluid. As a result, the contents of the stomach cannot empty quickly enough, and the athlete will experience side effects.

The types of carbohydrate that are available on the market today include sugars such as sucrose, fructose, and glucose. To supply higher amounts of carbohydrate for training and competition, carbohydrate sources such as maltodextrin, waxy maize starch, and superstarch have also been developed and formulated into sports drinks. These forms of carbohydrate have a lower osmolality. The osmolality of a drink is determined by the amount and type of carbohydrate and the amount of other particles such as electrolytes, sweeteners, and protein. The higher a drink's osmolality, the more difficult it is for the drink to leave the stomach. In comparison to drinks made up solely of sugars, maltodextrin, waxy maize, and superstarch can provide a significantly greater amount of carbohydrate in the same amount of fluid. In addition, carbohydrate such as superstarch has been shown to prevent gastrointestinal distress and help maintain a more desirable blood glucose profile, which is important for optimal performance. An athlete's energy needs and personal taste preferences will determine what is chosen to take in during training and competition.

Timeline

Athlete 1
Sport: Gymnastics
Sport requirements: Athletes are of light weight and have a low body-fat percentage and a high percentage of lean body mass.
Special concerns: The goal is to maintain muscle mass and decrease body fat.

- **More than 2 hours before:** A low-glycemic carbohydrate-based meal that provides an appropriate caloric dose based on estimations of energy flux

- **Less than 2 hours before:** Possibly a low-glycemic carbohydrate-based snack or beverage that provides an appropriate caloric dose based on estimations of energy flux

- **Less than 1 hour before:** A low-glycemic carbohydrate-based beverage with at least .5 grams of carbohydrate per kilogram of body weight

- **During:** Nothing

- **Immediately after:** A low-glycemic carbohydrate-based beverage that contains at least .5 grams of carbohydrate per kilogram of body weight and some whey protein or essential amino acids

- **Within 2 hours:** A low-glycemic carbohydrate-based meal that provides an appropriate caloric dose based on estimations of energy flux

- **More than 2 hours after:** Possibly a low-glycemic carbohydrate-based snack or beverage that provides an appropriate caloric dose based on estimations of energy flux

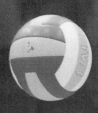

In team sports, players need to maintain strength and power endurance, as well as technical skill, throughout a match.

Protein Intake During Training and Competition

Protein is a food source that takes a longer amount of time to digest. As a result, most athletes do not take in protein during training unless participating in a sport that does not require high-intensity movements and that has long training sessions (>3 hours). Protein intake during training and competition revolves around either snacks and meals during an extended competition or the use of protein to prevent mental (a.k.a. central) fatigue.

Protein can greatly assist in controlling the glycemic response of a snack or meal. When athletes are training or competing all day long, keeping blood glucose stable, along with eating foods low in residue, is important. A meal made up of one-quarter to one-third protein consumed 2 hours before the start of training or competing will help minimize spikes in blood glucose. Amino acids added to fluids may also assist in this process, especially within an hour before competition. For athletes in technical sports or who must go through repeated rounds of competition in the same day, having stable blood glucose is very important.

Athletes engaged in all-day competition may find amino acids such as tyrosine or the branched-chain amino acids (leucine, isoleucine, and valine) to be beneficial in minimizing mental (central) fatigue and maintaining cognitive function. The central fatigue theory is related to the neurotransmitter serotonin. Serotonin makes a person feel relaxed and sleepy. Increases in this neurotransmitter are thought to be a result of more tryptophan, the amino acid that serotonin comes from, crossing the blood–brain barrier. When serotonin causes mental fatigue, this in turn can cause muscular fatigue, decrease focus, and thus limit performance. Tryptophan is thought to increase as a result of consumption of foods high in the amino acid; a high fat intake, which causes tryptophan to be released into the blood; or a decrease in branched-chain amino acids in the blood. All of these would allow for increased transport of tryptophan through the blood–brain barrier. Mixing tyrosine and branch chain amino acids into a carbohydrate–electrolyte beverage to consume during competition and throughout the day is most common. This also helps ensure that hydration is being maintained, which is the most important factor in sustaining cognitive function. Sports requiring the controlled execution of skills and rapid reaction or decision making, such as archery, taekwondo, shooting, and boxing, can benefit from reduced mental fatigue.

Fat Intake During Training and Competition

Fat intake during training and competition has been shown to enhance performance only in endurance sports of prolonged duration. Fat intake from food sources typically causes gastrointestinal distress; however, medium-chain triglycerides (MCTs) can be easily absorbed and have been shown to be of benefit.

MCTs are a popular type of fat with athletes because they are used by the body as quickly as carbohydrate and skip the long metabolic pathways that longer-chain fats must go through. Most research supports the use of MCTs plus a carbohydrate source. In fact, one study found that less energy was expended during a cycling time-trial performance when using an MCT plus carbohydrate versus carbohydrate only. It was noted that the difference in energy use could be attributed to lower circulating lactate concentrations and a reduced accumulation of hydrogen ions. Consuming small amounts of MCTs with carbohydrate has also been found to increase concentrations of free fatty acids without reducing carbohydrate oxidation. Consuming higher amounts of MCTs with carbohydrate may spare muscle glycogen and shift the body into using more fat as energy, even at higher intensities. However, athletes must take care when using MCTs during training and competition. Large quantities of MCTs may cause diarrhea, so athletes should follow a lower dosing pattern when first trying MCTs plus carbohydrate. A ratio of 5:1 carbohydrate to MCTs has been recommended in research, and this can be accomplished by drinking 100 milliliters every 10 minutes of a 2-gram MCT to 10-gram carbohydrate mixture, 60 to 90 minutes before training or competition. MCTs can be used by athletes who have difficulty maintaining or gaining weight. In small doses, they can be an effective way to add more calories to the daily eating plan without contributing to body-fat gain.

Posttraining Nutrient Strategies

Recovery is one of the most important factors in the process of adapting to training. The intake of fuel within 45 minutes of training can help optimize the recovery of energy stores, which is important for repairing muscle and maintaining a healthy immune system in athletes. In addition, consuming frequent small meals that contain the appropriate distribution of carbohydrate, protein, and fat also optimizes delivery of energy to the body throughout the remainder of the day to improve recovery and other factors such as body composition, which is critical for successful performance.

Timeline

Athlete 2
Sport: 10K running
Sport requirements: Athletes should optimize the weight-to-power ratio and maintain a low level of body fat.
Special concerns: The goal is to improve the ability of the body to utilize fat as a fuel source.

- **More than 2 hours before:** A low-glycemic carbohydrate-based meal that provides an appropriate caloric dose based on estimations of energy flux
- **Less than 2 hours before:** A low-glycemic carbohydrate-based snack or beverage that allows for at least 1 gram of carbohydrate per kilogram of body weight
- **Less than 1 hour before:** Nothing
- **During:** Nothing
- **Immediately after:** A low-glycemic carbohydrate-based beverage that provides at least .5 grams of carbohydrate per kilogram of body weight and that contains 6 to 20 grams of whey protein or essential amino acids
- **Within 2 hours:** A low-glycemic carbohydrate-based meal that provides an appropriate caloric dose based on estimations of energy flux
- **More than 2 hours after:** Possibly a low-glycemic carbohydrate-based snack or beverage that provides an appropriate caloric dose based on estimations of energy flux

Overcoming Postworkout Procrastination

You may have heard of the 30- to 60-minute window of opportunity after a workout in regard to eating. During this time, the receptors on the body's cells are more sensitive to insulin and therefore will accept the nutrients you eat more efficiently. The window begins to close after you finish your workout; as the cell receptors become less sensitive to insulin, your opportunity to efficiently use the food you eat decreases.

From a practical perspective, it is best to shorten this window because some athletes are procrastinators. That is, when asked to eat and drink something within 30 to 60 minutes, some athletes will wait 60 to 90 minutes, and their opportunity to fully utilize the nutrients they eat is not ideal. Additionally, because postworkout nutrition is so important for replenishing glycogen and fluid stores, the sooner an athlete can take in nutrition after a quality training session, the better. The best way to execute this is to plan ahead. Athletes should bring a small snack with them if they have to travel to a training session or prepare the postworkout snack ahead of time if working out at home so they do not have to find the motivation to make something afterward.

Carbohydrate Intake After Training and Competition

Carbohydrates are needed immediately after training or competition in order to begin the glycogen restoration process. Because glycogen stores are used during exercise, supplying the body with sources of carbohydrate is of utmost importance so the athlete can recover glycogen stores faster and be ready for the next session. This is even more important after a prolonged training session, especially if a second training bout is scheduled for the day.

After the initial postworkout consumption of a carbohydrate and protein snack, it is beneficial for athletes not seeking weight loss to eat another 1.0 to 1.2 grams of carbohydrate per kilogram of body weight 2 hours after the initial carbohydrate feeding and repeat throughout the next 6 to 8 hours in 2-hour increments. This strategy will refill glycogen stores the fastest, typically within 12 to 16 hours instead of 24 hours. Choosing any combination of carbohydrate during this time is beneficial as long as the foods are less processed and refined. Ideas include carbohydrate-rich snacks and meals balanced with lean protein such as a lean turkey sandwich with tomato, lettuce, cucumbers, pickles, and mustard; a nonfat milk-based fruit smoothie; a bowl of whole-grain cereal with berries and skim milk; or oatmeal made with skim milk and raisins. The goal is to maximize glycogen repletion, so eating smaller snacks or meals is preferred over larger ones that fill you up so much that you cannot eat again in another 2 hours.

Protein Intake After Training and Competition

Protein intake in the timeline immediately after training or competition can be used to repair muscle and restore muscle glycogen. Up to 20 grams of protein has been proven beneficial in facilitating carbohydrate uptake by the muscles, believed to result from protein's effect on the interaction of insulin with carbohydrate. An athlete's body size, training duration and intensity, and need to manage body weight will determine how much protein and carbohydrate is taken in. Athletes must learn to relate the size of a posttraining recovery snack to the intensity of the exercise bout. This is best exemplified by comparing a technique session to a high-intensity training session. After a technique session, a simple snack such as a yogurt that provides 6 to 8 grams of protein is sufficient, whereas a recovery shake containing 20 grams of protein would be appropriate after a high-intensity training session.

This rule can also be applied to athletes who are in a weight-loss phase. Regardless of training intensity, since energy intake must be reduced, the size of the postexercise snack must also be reduced. Thus, after a high-intensity session, 6 to 8 grams of protein would be sufficient, and the snack after a technique session could be completely eliminated. For athletes who must monitor body weight closely, a key component is minimizing food intake in the 2 hours after a resistance training session. This is the critical time period for increasing muscle synthesis. Although it would take multiple days and a significant increase in caloric intake to increase body mass, genetically some athletes are predisposed to building muscle mass rather easily. Thus, these athletes must do everything possible to keep this from happening, particularly in sports where a light body mass is required.

The second opportunity to take in protein is a meal within 2 hours after training. Protein at this point can be used to facilitate weight control or minimize the glycemic response of a meal, or it can serve a more minimal role in making a meal palatable. For athletes seeking to control body weight, protein can be increased in a meal to provide satiety and slow the rate at which glucose enters the blood. This will help optimize body composition, create satiety, and send the appropriate signals to the brain that indicate blood glucose is stable, and thus signals for hunger are not initiated. When weight loss is desired, the combination of protein, fiber, and water can create a sensation of fullness for a prolonged period of time. Protein has also been shown to help sustain lean body mass and cause a greater amount of fat loss. This is thought to be a result of its inefficient breakdown process, and thus very little usable energy is consumed, which helps further create a caloric deficit.

Athletes who need to keep body weight up or significantly replenish carbohydrate stores should minimize the amount of protein consumed in the recovery meal. Although protein can be used to make a meal palatable, these athletes need to minimize the satiety component. For athletes needing to gain weight, they must continue eating to create a positive energy balance. Athletes who deplete carbohydrate stores must consume enough food to fully restore muscle glycogen. Athletes competing in tournaments with bouts of high-intensity exercise for several hours daily need to pay particular attention to glycogen replenishment. This is most frequently seen in team sports and strength and power-type technical sports such as tennis and badminton.

The other role of protein is to minimize the glycemic response of snacks taken in between meals. This is important when trying to optimize body composition. Protein should be included in any snack eaten more than an hour before training, and it should make up at least 25 percent of the caloric value of the snack. This not only helps minimize an overconsumption of carbohydrate and increased snacking but also aids in satiety and slows the rate at which food empties from the stomach, thus controlling the glycemic response.

Timeline

Athlete 3

Sport: Volleyball

Sport requirements: Height is considered an advantage for most positions, and body composition varies substantially between players. The focus for optimal competition is to be able to maintain strength, power, stamina, and technical skill.

Special concerns: The goal is to improve on-court stamina.

- **More than 2 hours before:** A low-glycemic carbohydrate-based meal that provides an appropriate caloric dose based on estimations of energy flux

- **Less than 2 hours before:** Possibly a low-glycemic carbohydrate-based snack or beverage that provides an appropriate caloric dose based on estimations of energy flux

- **Less than 1 hour before:** Low- to moderate-glycemic carbohydrate-based snack or beverage that allows for at least 1 gram of carbohydrate per kilogram of body weight

- **During:** A 4 to 6% carbohydrate–electrolyte beverage if the athlete demonstrates the need for energy supply

- **Immediately after:** A low-glycemic carbohydrate-based beverage that contains at least .5 grams of carbohydrate per kilogram of body weight and 6 to 20 grams of whey protein or essential amino acids

- **Within 2 hours:** A low-glycemic carbohydrate-based meal that provides an appropriate caloric dose based on estimations of energy flux

- **More than 2 hours after:** Possibly a low-glycemic carbohydrate-based snack or beverage that provides an appropriate caloric dose based on estimations of energy flux

Fat Intake After Training and Competition

It has been theorized that intramuscular triglycerides (IMTGs) provide an energy source during exercise. These fats, stored inside the muscle, can decrease during exercise; thus, some researchers have studied the replenishment of IMTGs in the posttraining period. Although it has been shown that a high-carbohydrate and low-fat diet in the posttraining period may not fully replenish IMTGs, and moderate carbohydrate increases the stores more effectively, it is still unknown how important replenishing IMTG stores really is in terms of affecting performance.

Table 6.1 **Nutrient Intake After Training**

Nutrient	Recommendation
Carbohydrate	.5-1.2 g/kg of body weight
Protein	10-25 g
Fluid	24 oz/lb (1.6 L per kg) of body weight lost
Sodium	Minimum 500 mg/L of fluid consumed

Minimizing the amount of fat consumed in the first hour after a training session is recommended; the focus should be on ingesting carbohydrate, protein, fluid, and sodium. Fat—particularly omega-3 and monounsaturated—should be consumed at regular meals and snacks to provide a balanced macronutrient profile thereafter. Table 6.1 summarizes the nutrients that should be consumed in the period after training.

Crossover Concept

The unique role of protein and fat may come into play when athletes attempt to train on low glycogen stores in order to create a training adaptation. As mentioned previously, recent studies suggest that training in a low-glycogen state may help increase endurance capacity by maximizing adaptations in the muscles' mitochondria. The crossover concept is based on what source of fuel the body is using at rest and during submaximal exercise. Recent research shows that the ability to oxidize fat is important for high-level performance, optimal body composition, and even health. Well-trained athletes have an increased ability to use fat as a fuel source, and this is beneficial when carbohydrate stores become limited during prolonged bouts of training or competition.

Aerobic training induces cellular changes that improve the body's efficiency in using macronutrients, specifically fat. Mitochondria, which produce ATP (energy), increase in size and number as a result of aerobic training. Changes also occur in the activity of enzymes in the mitochondria; these changes make the oxidation of fatty acids more efficient. This allows the body to use more available fats for energy to fuel exercise. During anaerobic training sessions when the need to supply energy is very high, the ability to maximize fat oxidation becomes important so the energy demands of the body can be met.

The oxidation of fat by the mitochondria is the main source of energy when exercise intensity is low. Because glycogen stores can deplete rather quickly (after about 2 to 3 hours of continuous training at moderate intensity), and carbohydrate supplementation cannot provide adequate energy for longer-distance training because of gastrointestinal distress, it is beneficial for athletes to try to teach the body to have greater **metabolic efficiency** in using fats as an energy source.

Aerobic training is important to induce positive cellular changes, but just as important is the quality of food eaten during certain times of the physical periodiza-

metabolic efficiency – The body's ability to use stored fat as fuel during exercise and preserve carbohydrate.

tion program. The well-known physiological principle of periodization can be used in understanding how the right macronutrient utilization combined with physical training can have an impact on metabolic efficiency. In today's society many people consume carbohydrate before and during training, regardless of the purpose the training bout is supposed to serve. During low to moderate training intensities, this will make the body inefficient at learning to use fat as a fuel source, not only during training but also at rest. An example of this can be seen in figure 6.1, which shows an athlete who does not have a crossover of carbohydrate and fat utilization.

Research shows that ingestion of carbohydrate in the hours leading up to exercise and during exercise will suppress fat oxidation. When athletes perform low to moderate exercise training in a fasted state or on low carbohydrate intake before training, it improves the use of fat as a fuel source and reduces the use of muscle glycogen stores. The example provided in figure 6.1 can be corrected by training the body in a low-carbohydrate state during training sessions of low to moderate intensity. After training in this manner for four to six weeks, athletes will have an improved ability to use fat at rest and during low to moderate work intensities (figure 6.2, p. 104). The crossover of fat and carbohydrate as a fuel source can now be seen and is what should be expected.

Macronutrient strategies to produce the effects seen in figure 6.2 can be applied in an acute and short-term fashion. The acute strategy consists of refraining from carbohydrate ingestion in the several hours leading up to training and consuming a low-glycemic diet throughout the day. This strategy is often applied throughout the year to low-intensity training sessions. A longer but shorter-term strategy to aggressively improve the use of fat and carbohydrate during submaximal training bouts is to perform three to five days of training in a low-glycogen state. Training in a low-glycogen state can be beneficial; however, the body must still receive some form of energy to assist in muscle repair and to help maintain mood state. Although fat can

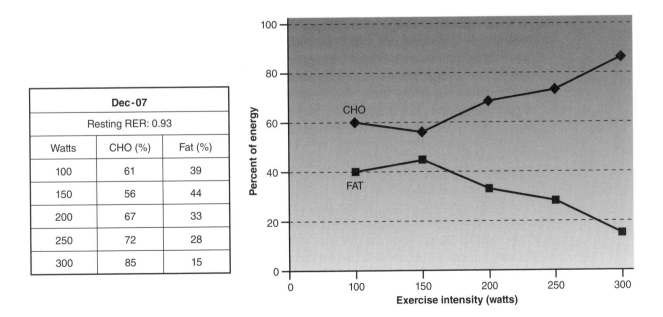

Dec-07		
Resting RER: 0.93		
Watts	CHO (%)	Fat (%)
100	61	39
150	56	44
200	67	33
250	72	28
300	85	15

Figure 6.1 This athlete demonstrates a high level of metabolic inefficiency as indicated by the high level of carbohydrate utilization and low level of fat utilization at very low exercise intensities. The goal for this athlete is to improve the ability to utilize fat as a fuel source at the lower exercise intensities and at rest. This will help the athlete improve body composition and delay glycogen depletion during prolonged exercise.

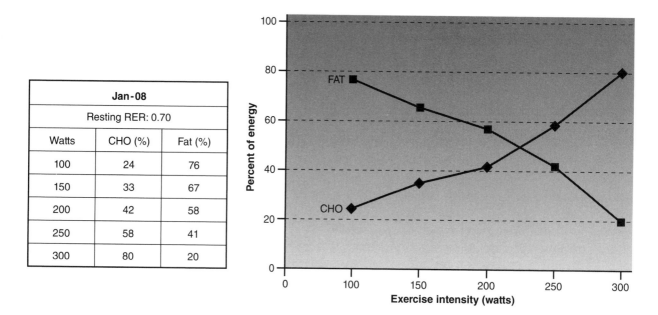

Jan-08		
Resting RER: 0.70		
Watts	CHO (%)	Fat (%)
100	24	76
150	33	67
200	42	58
250	58	41
300	80	20

Figure 6.2 After a one-month intervention of training without carbohydrate during low-, moderate-, and high-intensity exercise, as well as a change in nutritional intake to a diet that produces a low glycemic response, the athlete is now significantly more metabolically efficient at utilizing fat as a fuel source and minimizing the use of carbohydrate.

serve as an energy source, it has a higher caloric density than protein and can be far more difficult to digest. Thus, it is recommended to choose a balance of protein and fat when attempting to create a low-carbohydrate meal to keep glycogen low. When protein is the primary component of a meal, the timeline for food ingestion becomes altered. The best approach to consuming low-carbohydrate foods is to eat them in small amounts at frequent intervals. Eating based on hunger and satiety will most likely be preferred rather than eating at any given time intervals.

The crossover concept is important for athletes looking to improve the ratio of fat mass to muscle mass in the body. Regardless of body weight, it cannot be denied that improvements in performance are dependent on improving the ratio of power to muscle mass, and that as body composition improves, so does performance. Improving fat oxidation through the right combination of exercise training and food intake is the most effective way to assist athletes who are looking to improve their body composition and performance at the same time.

Conclusion

The macronutrients serve a very important role in the health and performance of athletes when consumption is centered on the training timeline and is designed to create a training adaptation. The key to manipulating macronutrient intake is basing the timing, type, and volume on the desired training adaptation. Strategies that help recover the body from training and that improve work capacity should be the focus of an athlete's nutrient timing program. This can include improving body composition, improving metabolic efficiency, and increasing power output through training.

Nutrition Periodization

Periodization involves changes in training volume and intensity throughout the year to induce positive physiological adaptations. Although there are many possible training cycles, this chapter focuses on the three basic ones used by most athletes and coaches: preseason, in-season, and off-season. The concept of physical periodization is well known and used by coaches and self-coached athletes. Formal and informal periodization plans have existed for decades and often include competition dates, training cycle goals and objectives, recovery modalities, physiology testing, and training camps.

Rationale for Periodization

Periodization can be defined as varying training throughout the year or years to manipulate volume and intensity to elicit positive physiological adaptations. Without periodization, an athlete would always be training for the same duration and at the same intensity, which could lead to overtraining and injury.

The periodization concept was introduced in the 1940s when Soviet sport scientists discovered that athletic performance was improved by altering the training stresses throughout the year rather than maintaining the same training plan month to month. This led to the division of an athlete's year into training cycles with differing physical stresses. The East Germans and Romanians further developed this concept by setting goals for the various periods, and periodization was born.

The traditional periodization concept separates a training program into specific cycles. The largest of these cycles is called a **macrocycle,** which is typically made up of the entire year (or four years for Olympic athletes). Within the macrocycle are smaller **mesocycles,** which can last several weeks to several months. The length depends largely on an athlete's goals, strengths and weaknesses, and any competitions. Each mesocycle can be divided into two or more smaller **microcycles** that are typically one week in length but could last up to four weeks. Microcycles are very specific and focus on daily exercise sessions. Most coaches and athletes use a series of terms to describe the cycles within a yearly periodization program. These typically include the following:

periodization – A process of structuring training into specific cycles over a year or several years.

macrocycle – A period of training that typically lasts from one to four years.

mesocycle – A period of training that typically lasts between 2 and 12 weeks.

microcycle – A period of training that typically lasts from several days to a week.

- Preseason, sometimes referred to as base. Athlete goals during this training cycle typically include improving cardiovascular fitness, general strength, technique, and flexibility.
- In-season, sometimes referred to as competition, build, or intensity. Athlete goals during this training cycle typically include improving power, force, sport-specific strength, economy, and tactics.
- Off-season, sometimes referred to as transition or recovery. Athlete goals during this training cycle typically include unstructured exercise to maintain fitness, prehabilitation, and rehabilitation. Athletes do not follow a structured training program during this time.

However, the best-constructed periodization plan is nothing without first considering the impact of other extrinsic factors that affect physical training and recovery. Nutrition certainly tops the list as one of the most important factors that contribute to physical training, but it often does not make it into a yearly periodization plan. It is certainly no secret that improperly fueling or hydrating the body can stop a training session short, significantly slow an athlete down, or in more serious instances, create an unplanned trip to the hospital. Periodizing an athlete's nutrition to support high and low training loads is paramount for sport development and attainment of peak performance. Table 7.1 shows some of the ways that nutrition and nutrient timing can support the basic annual periodization cycles for athletes.

Athlete Differences

Because of individual differences, the daily intake of macronutrients for athletes in different sports and even in the same sport will cover a large range. Although it is tempting to classify the lower ranges of the macronutrients for lower training levels and weight loss, this is not always the case, as will be described in each mesocycle's nutrition goals. The ranges provide a starting point and a foundation of knowledge to begin adapting the eating program to the training program. As previously mentioned, training load changes will largely dictate when and how to shift the distribution and timing of nutrients. Sports nutrition for athletes of all ages, abilities, and types has a strong science background, but when it comes to applying it to an athlete's specific needs, it becomes more of an art.

The macronutrient ranges for athletes cited in scientific research include 3 to 19 grams of carbohydrate per kilogram of body weight, 1.2 to 3.0 grams of protein per kilogram of body weight, and .8 to 3.0 grams of fat per kilogram of body weight. See table 7.2.

Table 7.1 **Nutrient Timing and Periodization**

Training cycle	Nutrition goals
Preseason (base)	• Timing, quantity, and quality of carbohydrate, protein, and fat
In-season (competition)	• Postworkout nutrition • Metabolic efficiency nutrition training
Off-season (transition)	• Energy control • Managing emotional eating

These ranges are large because of the many differences among athletes, body weight and body composition changes, and competition cycles. Each sport differs based on the duration of competition; the position played; and the weight classes in sports such as weightlifting, wrestling, and boxing.

Table 7.2 **Daily Ranges of Macronutrients for Athletes**

Macronutrient	g/kg of body weight
Carbohydrate	3-19
Protein	1.2-3.0
Fat	.8-3.0

Periodization and Nutrition Planning

Training load increases and decreases throughout the training year. With these changes come corresponding increases or decreases of stress on the body, which lead to different nutrient needs at certain times to handle and combat the stress responses to training. Nutrition periodization provides the required macro- and micronutrients at the right times during an athlete's training cycle to sustain health and thereby improve strength, speed, power, and endurance while helping to maintain a healthy immune system, body weight, and body composition. Stated simply, nutrition periodization supports training load changes so that athletes are able to achieve high-quality workouts and recover more quickly.

Athletes who are not nutritionally prepared before a quality training session will not receive the same positive physiological training adaptations as athletes who are prepared and place their nutrition on the top of their priority list.

Preseason

Before approaching nutrient needs and timing of the various training cycles, it is important to first have a clear understanding of the physical goals of each training cycle. This includes information relative to energy expenditure; frequency and focus of training sessions; and nutrition needs before, during, and after workouts.

The more popular physical goals for the preseason include improving strength, endurance, flexibility, and sport-specific technical and tactical skills. Weight loss and body composition may also be high on the priority list. Macronutrient ranges for this cycle should support physical training goals. If a hypertrophy (muscle building) stage is planned for strength training, the macronutrients would support this with higher calories and enough protein to remain in a positive protein balance. During a strenuous strength training session, protein stores can decrease, which may have a negative impact on improving lean muscle mass. Thus, timing protein before and after these types of training sessions is of utmost importance. In contrast, if weight loss or the improvement of body composition is the goal, a different nutrition plan focused on the proper timing of protein, healthy fat, and fiber-rich carbohydrate would be appropriate. Figure 7.1 on page 108 shows the overall dietary shifts appropriate for athletes seeking to maintain, gain, or lose weight in the preseason.

Daily Energy Balance

Remaining in a normal energy balance requires the management of carbohydrate, protein, fat, and alcohol intake with the energy expended through exercise, lifestyle, and resting metabolic rate. This somewhat delicate balance is maintained by accounting for

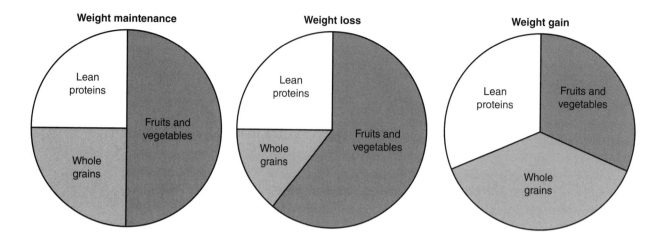

Figure 7.1 These charts show how food intake, by type of food, can be adjusted to meet the macronutrient needs of athletes seeking to gain or lose weight in the preseason.

the energy expenditure associated with the training cycle and the specific physiological goals as discussed earlier and matching it with the quantities of macronutrients consumed. There are many times in the early parts of the preseason where athletes stray out of energy balance. This is normally not due to the high energy expenditures from training but rather from justifying the need for more food. Athletes should be careful to match nutrition with training and thus remain in energy balance throughout this training cycle.

In general, carbohydrate intake in the preseason should range from 3 to 7 grams per kilogram of body weight (g/kg) for moderate-duration, low-intensity training (1 to 3 hours per day) and for weight loss or improving metabolic efficiency; range from 7 to 10 g/kg for moderate to heavy training (3 to 4 hours per day); and equal 10 or more g/kg for extreme training (4-plus hours per day). If a double is completed (e.g., a strength session and practice or two practices in one day), athletes should eat a minimum of 8 g/kg per day if they are not trying to lose weight. If weight loss is a goal, the lower end, 3 to 4 g/kg, is recommended as long as there is not much high-intensity or long-duration training.

The majority of carbohydrate consumption should be fruits and vegetables since they contain beneficial vitamins, minerals, antioxidants, and fiber. Whole grains can be eaten, but since most athletes do not consume enough fruits and vegetables, whole grains should be added after fruits and vegetables are consumed. A good goal is for an athlete to eat between 6 and 12 servings of fruits and vegetables per day. This goal can be easily accomplished by eating 1 or 2 fruits or vegetables at every meal and snack. Protein consumption can range from 1.2 to 2.0 g/kg for endurance-based athletes and from 1.6 to 3.0 g/kg for strength and power-based athletes. Endurance athletes normally do not need a high amount of daily protein unless weight loss is a goal, in which case protein can be used to improve satiety. The amount of fat remains relatively moderate at .8 to 1.3 g/kg. See table 7.3.

Table 7.3 **Preseason Daily Ranges of Macronutrients**

Macronutrient	g/kg of body weight
Carbohydrate	3-7 for 1-3 hours of training per day 7-10 for 3-4 hours of training per day 10 or more for 4+ hours of training per day
Protein	1.2-2.0 for endurance athletes 1.6-3.0 for strength and power athletes
Fat	.8-1.3

Staying hydrated can also have a positive effect on performance. Hydration guidelines that include a specific number of cups per day are outdated, as is assuming a portion of your body weight to determine the amount of water you drink. Hydration is very individual—some athletes may require more or less fluid for hydration based on many factors such as food intake, exercise frequency, intensity, time and type of exercise, sweat rate, geographical location, and environmental conditions. The best thing to do without having laboratory measurements such as urine-specific gravity tested every day is to base daily hydration on the color of urine and the frequency of urination. The color should be pale yellow to clear and not the color of apple juice. See chapter 2 for more information on assessing hydration status. Urinating frequently (every 2 to 3 hours) can also be a good marker of hydration status. One important thing to remember is that water is not the only way to meet daily fluid requirements. Athletes can also get water from other liquids or foods, especially those with a high water content such as fruits and vegetables.

The preseason is an ideal time of the training year for athletes to learn their hydration needs based on training duration and intensity. Depending on the training environment, sweat rates may not be as high as they will be in the next training cycle, where intensity is higher and duration is longer. Thus, learning the body's sweat response when first beginning a training program is extremely helpful, especially as athletes progress to the next, more demanding, training cycle. The preseason is also a good time for athletes to learn to drink when thirsty.

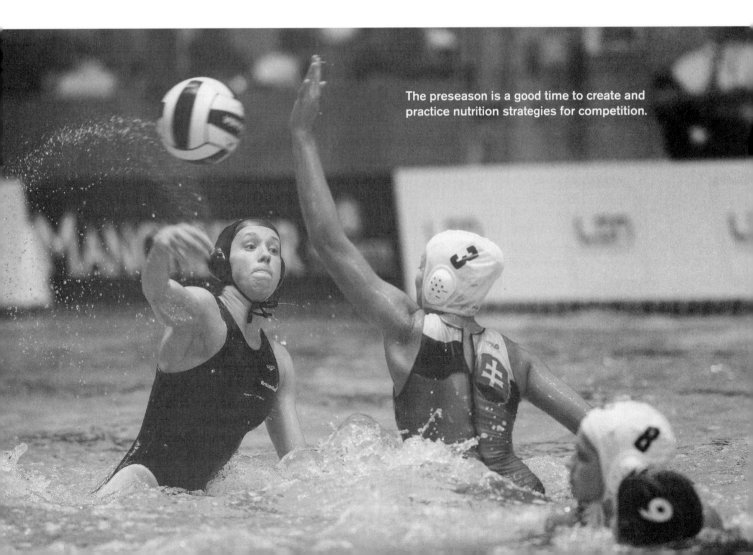

The preseason is a good time to create and practice nutrition strategies for competition.

Creating Nutrition Strategies for Competition

The preseason is a good time of the training year for athletes to learn how their bodies respond to certain foods before training and, more important, configure a plan of what to eat surrounding a training session. This can be considered "warming up the gut," which essentially means introducing certain foods before different training sessions to test the gut response. For example, an athlete who will be doing a training session on a bike may easily digest a bowl of oatmeal, but for an athlete running or undergoing a contact practice such as wrestling or football, this bowl of oatmeal may not sit well in the gut. Thus, specific nutrition strategies for before and during training can begin to be tested during the preseason.

Weight Loss

At some point in their athletic careers, most athletes will want to lose body fat. If an athlete aims to reduce fat mass during the preseason, it is important to establish a realistic timeline and goals along with the reasoning behind this weight or body-fat loss. Frequently athletes attempt to rapidly lose body weight or expect too great of a weight loss for the time frame they have in mind. As a result, their bodies' metabolisms will shut down in the process, and weight loss will come to a halt. To sustain training and achieve its benefits, most athletes should attempt to achieve weight loss at approximately 1 pound (.5 kg) per week and no more than 2 pounds (1 kg) per week.

Weight loss is best facilitated by creating a slight negative energy balance through increasing exercise and minimally restricting food intake. This can be accomplished by incorporating an additional 20 to 45 minutes of aerobic exercise (whether broken or continuous) five or six days per week and identifying three behavioral areas of food intake the athlete knows he can change, such as planning meals and snacks ahead of time, ensuring food is in the house, and going to the grocery store. One of the key aspects of successful weight loss is maintaining energy flux, specifically attempting to maintain the resting metabolic rate. This can be achieved by providing energy to the body in relation to when it is expended and then allowing the body to accept a small level of hunger in the latter part of the day.

Strategies for achieving a slight reduction in food intake include shifting the macronutrients, reducing food intake by 10 percent of typical intake, eating based on hunger, and using quantitative numbers to control food intake (e.g., a 250-calorie deficit). Should an athlete choose to use a quantitative method of inducing calorie restriction, it is important to assess starting food intake and energy expenditure levels. See chapter 2 for information on assessing energy intake and expenditure.

Regardless of the method used, most athletes will need to create a macronutrient shift, and athletes in aggressive resistance training programs should be careful to maintain a positive protein balance. Current recommendations suggest that most athletes will benefit from reducing their carbohydrate intake to 3 to 5 g/kg, although more may be required to support overall energy needs for athletes engaging in a hypertrophy-focused resistance training program. Because of the high satiety influence of protein, a higher amount of protein, from 1.8 to 2.5 g/kg, should be consumed, with special emphasis on higher-quality lean protein. Fat intake should remain low at .8 to 1.0 g/kg. See table 7.4.

Table 7.4 **Daily Ranges of Macronutrients for Preseason Weight Loss**

Macronutrient	g/kg of body weight
Carbohydrate	3-5
Protein	1.8-2.5
Fat	.8-1.0

Preseason Nutrition Training

This athlete is a collegiate water polo player who struggles with energy during training and competition. She and the coach wondered what could be done to improve her energy levels so she could optimize training to achieve her competitive ability. They know she is well conditioned for her sport and so looked to a nutritionist early in her preseason to see if energy supply might be an area they could improve. Review of the athlete's nutrition patterns revealed that she consumed a large majority of her caloric intake through high-glycemic carbohydrate. A test for resting metabolic rate showed that her body's choice of fuel even at rest was carbohydrate as demonstrated by a respiratory exchange ratio of .93. When blood glucose was tracked during training, it showed that her blood glucose levels would fall significantly and would continue to be low until a significant amount of carbohydrate could be ingested. This report indicates that her fatigue during competition was in part due to blood glucose levels becoming too low. During her nutrition review, it was also determined that the athlete struggled to eat before training or competing and that it was difficult for her to consume sufficient fluid when in training or competition.

Since the athlete was in her preseason training phase, it was a great time to begin changes in the macronutrient content of her nutrition intake. The new plan provided her with the same total caloric intake while creating a low to moderate glycemic response. This would help her body regulate blood glucose levels more steadily and help her body learn how to tap into her fat stores in order to supply more fuel efficiently. By the time this intervention was completed, the athlete was in her precompetition phase. This allowed for the other issue that arose during the nutrition consult to be addressed: consuming food and fluid before and during training.

Over the next four weeks, the athlete practiced taking in larger amounts of a carbohydrate–electrolyte beverage in the hour before training, and during training she took sips of fluid as frequently as possible and moved to gulps of fluid over the four-week period. This trained her stomach to handle fluid during exercise. The end result for the athlete was a high level of sustained energy during training by the time the competitive season started. This was backed by blood glucose values remaining steady during training and competition. In addition, a follow-up test for resting metabolic rate showed a new respiratory exchange ratio of .78, indicating the athlete had learned to use fat as a fuel source much more efficiently.

The ability to lose weight highly depends on the athlete's motivation, mental state, and history and methods of weight loss. One of the better weight-loss methods is to use the fullness factor (rather than count calories or grams of the macronutrients), sometimes referred to as high satiety, by combining good sources of lean protein with fiber-rich foods. This will maintain blood sugar levels, and the fullness factor combined with increasing the volume of aerobic training (for sports where this type of training is appropriate) will elicit the most beneficial type of weight loss for athletes.

Weight Gain

Athletes wishing to gain weight in the preseason face just as many challenges, if not more, as those seeking to lose weight. Common complaints from athletes who are not successful in gaining weight include not being able to eat enough throughout the day. This difficulty can be remedied through proper nutrient timing coupled with choosing high-quality nutrients. Table 7.5 shows daily macronutrient recommendations for athletes trying to gain weight.

Table 7.5 **Daily Ranges of Macronutrients for Preseason Weight Gain**

Macronutrient	g/kg of body weight
Carbohydrate	10 or more
Protein	1.8-2.5
Fat	1.0-1.3

Athletes trying to gain weight can have great success with shakes or smoothies made of lean protein sources such as milk or protein powders and carbohydrate sources such as fruit or fruit juices. A small amount of healthy oil such as canola, olive, or flax can be added for additional calories. Consuming protein with carbohydrate before and after strength training sessions is beneficial for maintaining a net protein synthesis rate and will help prevent protein breakdown during a weights session. Additionally, athletes who follow a very healthy, or "clean," diet consisting of higher-fiber foods from whole grains and fruits and vegetables, lean protein sources from meats and dairy products, and few or no refined and processed foods may have difficulty gaining weight since they will experience a high level of fullness. This type of eating works well for weight loss, but when it comes to weight gain, focusing on starchy foods a bit lower in fiber and reducing lean protein to promote more frequent hunger throughout the day are better strategies.

Eating Throughout Training Sessions

Having adequate fluid and glycogen stores is extremely important for being able to attain the physical goals of practice and training sessions. Most athletes do well by eating a small snack consisting of easy-to-digest carbohydrate and a small amount of protein and fat with adequate fluid. Of course this depends greatly on the sport. For example, triathletes usually have to find three different snacks that work before their three different sports, whereas single-sport athletes can usually have one or two go-to snacks. Good recommendations are liquid or semi-solid sources of calories such as a milk-based fruit smoothie, a banana with a small amount of peanut butter, or yogurt with fruit. A glass of water should be part of the snack if fluid isn't included. It is best to allow 1 to 3 hours between the snack and the training session, so preparation and planning are crucial.

Consuming fluid and calories during a practice or training session is highly variable based on the athlete, sport, environmental conditions, and breaks that coaches plan during practices. Although these can be ever changing, there are a few general recommendations that athletes can follow and customize to their specific preseason practice or training session.

Staying hydrated is extremely important throughout training. Current recommendations include drinking .07 to .10 ounces of fluid per pound (4.7 to 6.6 ml/kg) of body weight 4 hours before training and an additional .04 to .10 ounces of fluid per pound (2.7 to 6.6 ml/kg) of body weight 2 hours before training if the urine is not pale yellow in color.

In general, carbohydrate consumption recommendations can range from 30 to 90 grams (120 to 360 calories) per hour of training. Of course, this will depend greatly on the sport and athlete and whether or not frequent breaks are taken. For example, cross country runners are infamous for not drinking or consuming anything with calories during runs. In contrast, some team-sport athletes may have many opportunities to consume carbohydrate during training but may choose not to since it is does not mimic competition conditions. Soccer is one example of this; frequent breaks are taken throughout practice, but during a match, there is only one opportunity to refuel, and most players cannot consume a high amount of carbohydrate during halftime because of the short duration of the break and the inability to process a large amount of food immediately before returning to high-intensity exercise.

Because such a large range exists, the take-home message is that during higher-quality training sessions, defined as longer than 2 to 3 hours or of very high intensity, some carbohydrate is needed to maintain mental concentration as well as fuel the working muscles. Keep in mind that sometimes throughout the training year, carbohydrate may not be needed during workouts and may even prevent the body from improving fat usage during certain exercise intensities. This will be discussed later in the chapter.

If you are training up to 90 minutes at a moderately high intensity, try consuming up to 50 grams (200 calories) of carbohydrate per hour. For training more than 2 hours at submaximal exercise, consume up to 60 grams (240 calories) per hour. Depending on your digestive system, you can choose a solid or liquid form of carbohydrate. Remember that during low- to moderate-intensity exercise, blood flow to the stomach is fairly adequate, which means you should be able to choose easily digestible carbohydrate such as lower-fiber energy bars or bagels. During higher-intensity exercise, blood flow to the stomach is lower, which means you should consume more liquids, semi-solids (such as bananas), and energy gels. Consuming fluid during training sessions will help maintain fluid balance, and drinking between 3 and 8 ounces (90 and 240 ml) of fluid every 15 to 20 minutes is recommended.

If more than one training session is done throughout the day, postworkout nutrition becomes crucial, and although it will depend on the mode of the next exercise bout (e.g., aerobic versus anaerobic work), athletes should begin the repletion of nutrients immediately after the first session and introduce a small to moderate amount of nutrition in a steady state until their next training session. Of course, nutrition before the first workout is very important because a good breakfast allows athletes to replace some of the nutrients that are used during sleep.

In-Season

During the competitive season, nutrient timing becomes even more important for athletes because games, races, and matches become more frequent. This puts more stress on the body, and recovering from competitions is a key to optimal performance. It is important for athletes to develop and follow a nutrition warm-up. That is, they should use the information gained during the preseason to determine which foods in what quantities worked before high-quality training sessions. It is likely that these food combinations will work the same before competitions, but it is best to try these feeding strategies in competition simulations. Athletes often practice their nutrition during training sessions or practices that do not mimic their predicted competition intensity. Remember that as intensity of exercise increases, the body's ability to digest food decreases.

For most athletes, improving sport-specific strength, power, force, speed and economy, and competition tactical and technical knowledge is the main goal. During this mesocycle, athletes will burn more calories through training; therefore, active weight loss is not recommended since the quality of training may suffer. That said, some athletes will experience passive weight loss, or weight loss due to increased intensity, which correlates into a higher energy expenditure. The biggest mistakes are made during this time of the season by not eating frequently, making poor-quality food choices that do not support the energy needed to sustain higher-intensity training sessions, and taking hydration for granted by not staying hydrated throughout and before training sessions.

Overall, most of the in-season macronutrient guidelines follow similar, if not exact, patterns to that of the preseason because the body is adapted to the timing and quantity of foods and beverages. One factor that may change significantly is the quality of calories consumed. Because of the stress associated with competitions and the repeated nature of higher-intensity training sessions, more rapidly absorbed carbohydrates are beneficial, as is the practice of using sports drinks for hydration, carbohydrate–electrolyte, and in some cases, protein purposes. The basic rule of thumb is that most of the gastrointestinal conditioning of various foods and their quality and quantities should have been close to finalized during the preseason. The worst thing to do during the competition season is to drastically alter the nutrition plan. Small deviations that account for fitness level, environment, or duration of competitions are fine and must be both accounted for and implemented. It is the large nutrition changes that should be avoided.

Carbohydrate intake is similar to the preseason, but because athletes will most likely be doing at least two or more high-intensity training sessions or competitions each week, athletes should choose the higher end of the recommended range of carbohydrate per kilogram of body weight. This concept is termed *microcycle periodization*—that is, adjusting daily nutrient intake with daily training load. It is very unlikely for athletes to work at the same volume and intensity each day of the week, so it is beneficial to eat according to these fluctuations. On off days or light days, athletes should choose the lower end of the range as long as they have eaten adequate carbohydrate after quality training sessions on previous days. This lets the athletes remain weight stable by not overconsuming calories on days of lower energy expenditure and will improve recovery times by getting the right nutrients on the days of higher intensity or longer duration.

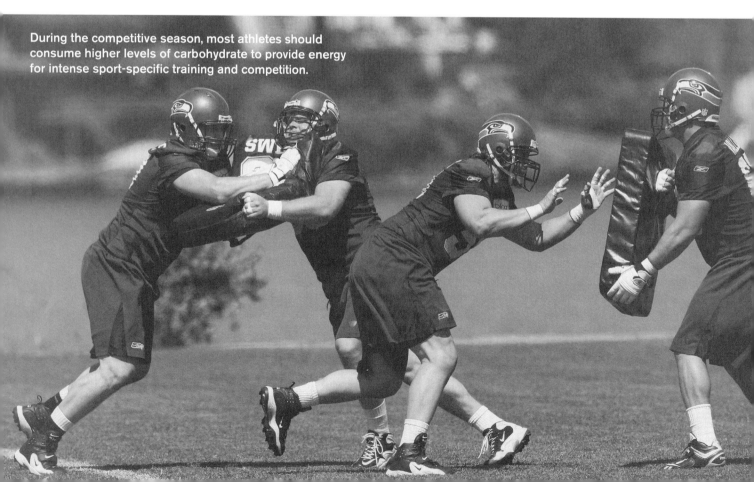

During the competitive season, most athletes should consume higher levels of carbohydrate to provide energy for intense sport-specific training and competition.

The range for protein can remain similar to the preseason or increase slightly if there are more frequent intense speed training sessions and strength training. Remember, balancing and maintaining protein stores that can be depleted during these types of training sessions is the goal.

The range for fat is also similar to the preseason cycle with the exception of training for ultraendurance races. Athletes falling into this category will likely require a small amount of additional fat in their eating programs because of the higher energy loss from longer-duration training sessions. Fat is more energy dense and will assist these athletes in remaining in energy balance more effectively. Of course, healthier fats such as polyunsaturated (specifically omega-3) and monounsaturated fats should make up most of the fat intake, with very minimal amounts of saturated fats.

No matter the training cycle, hydration recommendations are fairly consistent. Remember to factor in the environment and travel, both domestic and international, as these can have significant impacts on hydration protocol implementation.

Eating Throughout Training Sessions

Most of the macronutrient recommendations for before, during, and after workouts and competitions are similar to that of the preseason for the reasons mentioned previously. However, the one significant change pertains to carbohydrate intake.

Newer research has found that the body can absorb more carbohydrate under certain conditions. This can mean huge benefits for athletes who expend a high amount of calories during training or competition because it may allow them to fuel better and delay malnutrition longer. Based on this new research, the recommended high end of the carbohydrate intake range is 90 grams per hour versus the previous 60 grams. However, it is important to realize that eating upwards of 90 grams of carbohydrate per hour is not easy and is not recommended for all athletes. For smaller, female, and team-sport athletes where most of the training and competitions consist of short bursts of speed, power, and strength, a range of 30 to 50 grams of carbohydrate per hour is recommended. For athletes training at near-maximal intensity for more than 2 hours, a 50- to 70-gram range is recommended, and 60 to 90 grams per hour is recommended for athletes competing at submaximal intensity levels for greater than 6 hours. The easiest way for athletes to ensure they are consuming enough carbohydrate is through liquid sources, such as sports drinks, since they are easier to digest during exercise.

Off-Season

For most athletes who have an off-season, this time of the training year is a time of rest, recovery, and rejuvenation, at least for a couple of weeks. Because the physical goals differ significantly from the preseason and in-season, this is the cycle during the year where most nutrition mistakes are made that lead to unnecessary body-weight and body-fat gains. The goals for athletes during this cycle should therefore include controlling the amount of energy consumed and improving metabolic efficiency. This is described in more detail in chapter 6, but in brief, teaching the body to use its internal fat stores throughout a wide range of intensities is extremely beneficial, as this can fuel exercise and thus preserve internal carbohydrate stores. Because the body has an almost unlimited amount of fat stores and an extremely limited amount of carbohydrates stores, it is very beneficial to teach the body to become more metabolically efficient. This not only has a carbohydrate-sparing effect but can also make a significant impact on body composition. Utilizing more internal fat stores can have a positive correlation with reducing body fat, and during the off-season, this could give an athlete a better advantage going into the preseason conditioning program.

During the competitive season, the body's energy demands are increased because of higher-intensity training and competing; caloric intake is therefore typically higher to match the high expenditure. Although this is nutrition periodization at its finest, it is very difficult for athletes to "flip the switch" when it comes to decreasing food intake, even though training volume is much lower. A nutrition change of this magnitude requires a behavior change, and this could take weeks to months. During the first year of implementing a solid nutrient timing and nutrition periodization plan, there are many things to learn. This first off-season using these concepts will be more difficult than future years, but it is certainly not impossible to implement a few simple off-season nutrition principles.

One of the easiest to begin with is the elimination of all nutrition supplements that provide calories. Products such as energy bars, gels, sports drinks, and powders are simply not necessary during this time of the year. Remember that the primary goal is energy control, and these products become roadblocks to most athletes' nutrition goals in the off-season. This simple measure will help prevent the unnecessary weight gain that often plagues athletes. However, an exception is strength and power athletes who are trying to increase mass during the off-season. The recommendation for these athletes to ensure they consume a high number of total calories, including sufficient carbohydrate and protein.

The second goal—improving metabolic efficiency—is discussed in more detail in chapter 6, but in brief, focusing on a more balanced daily nutrition program consisting of lean protein, healthy fat, and fruits and vegetables will provide a metabolic shift of teaching the body to utilize more of its fat stores by keeping blood sugar more stable. This is an ideal scenario for athletes as they approach the preseason. In fact, daily carbohydrate intake decreases to 3 to 4 g/kg, with most of the emphasis on fruits and vegetables and less on whole grains and healthier starches. Protein, specifically lean sources, can range from 1.5 to 2.3 g/kg if used for satiety purposes and to prevent overeating. Fat remains low at 1.0 to 1.2 g/kg, with the emphasis on omega-3 fats, and hydration goals are focused on noncalorie beverages that will not provide unnecessary calories during this time of lower energy expenditure. See table 7.6.

When athletes exercise during the off-season, nutrition goals become much simpler. A light, balanced meal or snack will provide the body with more than enough energy for the session. During exercise, 3 to 8 ounces (90 to 240 ml) of water every 20 to 30 minutes, and possibly small amounts of electrolytes (500 mg/L), is all that is required to maintain hydration status. Because exercise sessions will not come close to depleting glycogen stores, taking supplemental carbohydrate is not necessary during this cycle. Postexercise nutrition focuses on replenishing hydration stores by drinking 24 ounces (720 ml) of water with at least 500 mg/L of sodium immediately after the session. A light snack or meal that includes a good source of carbohydrate, lean protein, and a small amount of fat will also suffice. Remember, the main goal of this cycle is to control energy intake, and the easiest way to do this is by forgoing unneeded calories consumed during exercise sessions.

Table 7.6 **Off-Season Daily Ranges of Macronutrients**

Macronutrient	g/kg of body weight
Carbohydrate	3-4
Protein	1.5-2.3
Fat	1.0-1.2

Conclusion

Combining a sound nutrient timing regimen with a yearly periodized nutrition plan allows athletes to enhance health, improve performance, and manipulate body weight and body composition based on their sport and training cycle needs. Care should be taken in the planning and preparation of a nutrition program, just as is typically done with the training program. Allowing nutrition periodization to support an athlete's physical periodization will lead to positive physical adaptations resulting in optimal performance.

Long-Term Athlete Development and Periodization

This female taekwondo athlete was 15 years old and had been participating in the sport for 6 years when she originally began to consider her nutrition. She had already achieved the status of being the top national competitor in her weight class at the junior and senior level.

The sport of taekwondo is a Korean martial art that is classified by weight categories. Athletes are required to make weight on the day before competition and have approximately 18 hours from the time of weigh-in until they compete. Sparring at the competitive level is full contact and allows fighters of all belt levels to compete in sparring. A match takes place between two competitors in an area measuring 8 square meters. Each match consists of 3 2-minute rounds of contact, with a 1-minute rest between rounds. Points are awarded for techniques that are delivered to the legal scoring areas of the hogu (chest protector). At the end of three rounds, the competitor with the most points wins the match. In the event of a tie, a fourth sudden-death over-time round is held to determine the winner. In a tournament, the successful athlete may compete in up to five rounds within the day. The amount of time between rounds can be anywhere from 2 hours at the start of the day's competition and no more than 30 minutes by the end of the day.

This athlete's primary goal for the year was to make the world championship team at the fin weight class (46 kg; 101.4 lb). Over the next two years, the athlete was planning to move up one weight class to fly (49 kg; 108.0 lb), as it is competed at the Olympic Games. The goal was to make the Olympic Team. To do this, the athlete and her coach had set goals to increase speed, strength, and power, all of which are critical athletic characteristics for being a competitive taekwondo athlete.

Before this, the athlete had not paid any attention to what or when she ate. Mom had tried to cook healthy meals, but because of a hectic work schedule, the family frequently ate out for dinner. There was also a large supply of processed snack foods kept in the house. It was a habit of the entire family to snack on these foods continuously throughout the day. There were no set times for meals, and the purpose of eating was not known. Frequently, the family was very hungry before a meal was even considered, and this further promoted quick snacks from processed foods. At meal time, the family ate quickly and without any conscious decisions about when their bodies signaled they were full and satisfied.

BACKGROUND OF SPECIFIC ISSUES RELATIVE TO NUTRITION

In the past years, this athlete's body weight had always naturally been at her competitive weight class, and so this was not a concern; however, recently the athlete, her coach, and her parents all became aware that the athlete's height and weight were continuing to increase and she had not yet reached puberty. She was 5 feet 3.5 inches (161 cm) and 106 pounds (48 kg). With an increased focus on becoming a high-level competitor, this athlete had realized that she must focus on how nutrition can help manage body weight appropriately and support not only how her body was growing but also the desired training adaptations. A once-monthly plan was put in place to monitor height, weight, body composition, and performance testing. Performance testing included tests for power, speed, and agility (vertical jump, long jump, 30-meter acceleration, and octagon multidirectional agility).

NUTRITION GOAL

Her main goal was to make the Olympic team and eventually become an Olympic and world championship medalist. To achieve her goal, the athlete needed to determine the weight class that was best for her to compete at while maintaining and continuing to improve her speed, power, and agility in combination with the technical skills of taekwondo.

NUTRITION PLAN

The first step was to make the athlete aware of what she was eating, how frequently, how much she was drinking, and her instinctive eating signals. Three simple goals were set after realizing that each day she consumed only five glasses of water, two fruits, and no vegetables and ate only when hunger signals were high at 5 to 6 hours after the last meal or snack. Her initial goals were as follows:

1. Increase fluid consumption to eight glasses of water daily, with at least one being consumed at every meal or snack.

2. Consume a meal or snack every 3 hours, eating until full and satisfied.

3. Increase fruit and vegetable intake by one serving every three days until she was eating six servings total on a daily basis.

The timeline shows a sample daily meal plan to accomplish this athlete's goals.

⏱ Timeline

Sample Daily Meal Plan
Drink eight glasses of water, spread throughout the day.

• **Pretraining snack:** Whole-grain bread with almond butter and banana

• **Posttraining snack:** Low-glycemic carbohydrate and protein recovery beverage and dark chocolate

• **Breakfast:** High-fiber cereal, skim milk, and berries

• **Lunch:** Mozzarella and tomato salad with couscous

• **Snack:** Greek yogurt, granola, agave nectar, seeds, mango

• **Dinner:** Red chicken curry (meal included vegetables)

• **Dessert or snack:** Spiced fruit with vanilla frozen yogurt

After a month of consistent practice, the athlete's height and weight had increased to 5 feet 5 inches (165 cm) and 112 pounds (51 kg). Body composition had stayed consistent, and there were no significant changes in her performance tests. Most important, speed and agility had not decreased despite an increase in body weight. With team trials for the world championships only a month away, it was decided that she would compete in the fly division rather than fin weight. New goals were set for after the team trials:

1. Begin learning to cook.

2. Match fluids to sweat rate and daily body needs.

3. Learn the functionality of foods, and consume them appropriately in the developed timeline.

Two months after the team trials, she had grown another inch (2.5 cm) and weight had again increased by two pounds, and goals had to be set to ensure her body weight did not get too high for making weight at the world championships. This was facilitated by three strategies:

1. She replaced half the calories coming from starches with calories from fruit with good fiber content.

2. Instead of 2 percent milk before and after weight training, she drank skim milk an hour before the start of training.

3. Her postexercise recovery drink after taekwondo training sessions was cut in half.

A key aspect of going to the world championships was preparing for what foods she may or may not have access to. She purchased a hot pot, and the nutritionist made up a list of key food items for her to take with her. This included sports drinks; carbohydrate and protein powder; favorite competition snack foods; and packets of chicken, soup, and beans and rice mixture that she could easily make.

Once the world championships were over for the year, she took a month off with the goal of seeing if her body would continue to grow. After this regeneration period, she was 5 feet 6 inches (168 cm) and 118 pounds (53 kg) and had not begun menstruation. This was a clear indicator that her body was still going to grow, and an increase in calories was needed to continue supporting her growth. Looking to the future, it was decided that the best weight class for her to compete in given the competition at Olympic trials would be the weight class that required her to be above 57 kg (125.7 lb) and no higher than 67 kg (147.7 lb). Until the Olympics, she would fight at the weight class closest to her natural body weight.

Competing at a higher body weight required that she begin to increase muscle mass at approximately 1 pound (.5 kg) per month over the next year. Since growth would naturally be occurring anyway, only one change was initiated. A greater amount of fat was included in her snack before and after weight training, which has been shown to help increase muscle synthesis. This increase came from a variety of fats, from nut butters, dairy products, avocados mixed in with a meat and carbohydrate source, olives, hummus, and any combination that would provide the healthy fats plus protein and a carbohydrate source.

Over the next year an important aspect of this athlete's development was not only an increase in muscle mass but also an improvement in agility, speed, and power scores. These measures demonstrated the effects of training properly and that she was adapting to the increase in body weight. From this point forward, the goal was to stay consistent and to define success based on process goals that she and her coach had set for improving her chances of making the team. Measurement of body weight and composition was then necessary only to further evaluate performance testing and thus was done only at the end of a training cycle. This helped the athlete keep a positive and healthy outlook about weight management. She eventually became 5 feet 10 inches (178 cm) and 154 pounds (70 kg) before making the Olympic team and competed in the over 57 kg and under 67 kg weight class.

EIGHT

Nutritional Supplementation

In today's society, most people consume some form of nutritional supplement. In the athletic setting, supplements are not uncommon, and most athletes are looking for the next latest and greatest product to enhance training and performance. It cannot be argued that supplements have the potential to enhance performance; however, what can be highlighted is that the inappropriate use of supplements does not bring benefits to an athlete but rather can cost an extreme amount of money, deter performance, and at times have unforeseen consequences. Thus, the goal must be to design and implement a timing system for supplement ingestion so that the desired training or nutrition benefit is received. Athletes who learn to use supplements strategically can enhance performance.

In this chapter, three different classifications of nutritional supplements are addressed: dietary supplements, sport supplements, and ergogenic aids. Most athletes believe that nutritional supplements can enhance performance. Dietary supplements such as multivitamins, calcium, and iron are often taken as an insurance policy, to help prevent or treat an injury, to assist in healing during an illness or disease, or to compensate for inadequate food intake. Sport supplements are frequently used to supply fuel before, during, and after training sessions. They are also frequently used in place of food when athletes are not prepared to cook or when athletes believe sport supplements can assist in weight control, enhance physical appearance, or substitute for the nutrients found in food. **Ergogenic** aids are commonly used as a means to enhance performance through an increase in work capacity. The sidebar provides a list that classifies supplements addressed in this chapter.

ergogenic –
Performance enhancing.

Evaluating Supplements

The first step in identifying the nutritional supplements that are right for any athlete is to determine whether or not research supports the claims made about their potential effects. The following is a list to help determine if a supplement may be worth trying:

1. Does it promise quick improvements in health or physical performance?
2. Does it contain a secret ingredient or formula?

Common Supplements and Ergogenic Aids

DIETARY SUPPLEMENTS

Multivitamins

Iron

Calcium

Zinc

Antioxidants

Glucosamine and chondroitin

Omega-3 fatty acids

B-complex vitamins

Fiber

SPORT SUPPLEMENTS

Preworkout beverage

During-workout beverage

Postworkout beverage

Electrolytes

Whey and casein protein

Soy protein

ERGOGENIC AIDS

Caffeine

Creatine

Sodium bicarbonate

Beta-alanine

Glycerol

Phosphagen

Colostrum (bovine)

Beta-hydroxy-beta-methylbutyrate (HMB)

Amino acids

3. Can you recognize the ingredients or easily learn what they are intended for in the physical body?

4. Is there only anecdotal evidence or testimonials to support the claims made regarding improvements in health or physical performance?

5. Are the claims supported by substantial research indicating improvements in health or physical performance?

6. Who is advertising or selling the product? Celebrities? Star athletes? The person who invented the product?

7. Does the product potentially exaggerate that a nutrient frequently found in foods can significantly enhance performance?

8. What is the cost of the supplement in relation to obtaining the same nutrient from foods?

9. Do the benefits sound too good to be true?

The sidebar on page 124 shows an example of how these questions could be applied to a supplement. This is not a real company or supplement name, but similar products are on the market.

The second step in identifying appropriate nutritional supplements is to determine where the product is produced. Quality assurance in the production of nutritional supplements continues to be a concern. As a result, it is important to identify products that carry a seal of approval such as USP (United States Pharmacopeia) on the label, are made by well-known food and drug manufacturers that follow good manufacturing practices (GMPs), are supported by research, and make only accurate and appropriate claims. In addition, it is highly recommended that the company be able to provide a **certificate of analysis** for the product as well as allow independent laboratories to test for the purity and quality of the product.

Several programs have been put in place to ensure that companies produce their products under GMP guidelines. The National Nutritional Foods Association (NNFA) in the United States has an alliance with NSF International, which has a product certification program. Under the guidelines provided by the NNFA, a product is listed as produced under GMP guidelines only if the company is a member of the organization and has passed a raw materials guarantee for each batch of product that is produced. NSF International serves to test any product that is part of the NNFA. As a result, athletes can be guaranteed that a product is pure and contains the quality ingredients that it claims. In addition to these measures, three other resources are available to independently test nutritional supplements. ConsumerLab.com and Informed Choice both test nutritional supplements for banned substances and will identify whether or not products have been safely screened for contamination. They can provide the batch or lot number that has been tested. The United States Food and Drug Administration also has a program in place to identify products manufactured under GMP programs and tests products for harmful and banned substances; however, not all supplements are tested by the FDA.

Dietary Supplements

Dietary supplements encompass the micronutrients that most athletes take, either for known deficiencies or as insurance policies. They are typically taken throughout the entire training year, although some are phased in and out depending on an athlete's needs and deficiency states. Popular supplements that are part of this category include multivitamins, iron, calcium, zinc, antioxidants, glucosamine and chondroitin, omega-3 fats, B-complex vitamins, and fiber.

Vitamins are metabolic catalysts that regulate chemical reactions within the body. Most vitamins are chemical substances that the body does not manufacture, so it is important to obtain them from foods. Minerals are elements obtained from foods that combine in many ways to form structures of the body (e.g., calcium in bones) and regulate body processes (e.g., iron in red blood cells transports oxygen).

Multivitamins

Most people who take multivitamins do so as an insurance policy against deficiencies in vitamins and minerals. There are many multivitamins available on the market, and they frequently contain megadoses of their ingredients, which should be avoided. Rather, it is best to purchase a multivitamin that contains no more than the recommended dietary allowance (RDA) for each of the vitamins and minerals listed. Multivitamins can come with or without iron. When determining whether or not to choose a multivitamin that contains iron, it is best to consider whether an athlete is at risk of developing any type of iron deficiency. Calcium, which is often included in multivitamins, can inhibit the absorption of iron. Iron and copper compete because they use the same transporter in the body. If an athlete needs to ensure adequate iron stores, it is best to choose an individual iron supplement and a multivitamin without iron. The iron should be taken separately from the multivitamin to ensure the best chance for absorption.

certificate of analysis – A document that reports and certifies the test results of a product.

dietary supplement – A product that contains substances such as vitamins, minerals, foods, botanicals, and amino acids and is intended to supplement the usual intake of these substances. Dietary supplements are found in pill, tablet, capsule, powder, or liquid form and are meant to be taken by mouth.

Critically Evaluating a Supplement

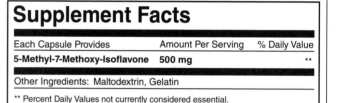

Max-Pro Methoxy Tech 500

- Increase nitrogen retention
- Increase $\dot{V}O_2$max (more endurance)
- Increase strength
- Decrease body fat
- Improve stamina and libido
- Surpass your genetic potential

Max-Pro Methoxy Tech 500 is a nonhormonal anabolic and anticatabolic agent. This powerful flavone has shown to increase protein synthesis and speed muscles' recovery from exercise. 5-Methyl-7-Methoxy-Isoflavone, the official chemical name, is an all-natural ingredient that was discovered and patented by a secretive company decades ago. It wasn't until 1996 that this ingredient was made available on the free market. Dozens of studies uncovered performance-improving benefits that must be experienced to be believed. Just $60 for a one-month supply.

Max-Pro Methoxy Tech 500
- Increase nitrogen retention
- Increase $\dot{V}O_2$max (more endurance)
- Increase strength
- Decrease body fat
- Improve stamina and libido
- Surpass your genetic potential

Supplement Facts

Each Capsule Provides	Amount Per Serving	% Daily Value
5-Methyl-7-Methoxy-Isoflavone	**500 mg**	**

Other Ingredients: Maltodextrin, Gelatin

** Percent Daily Values not currently considered essential.

Study the label and the promotional claims provided for this supplement. How could the evaluation questions help an athlete or coach make a decision about the value of this supplement?

1. *Does it promise quick improvements in health or physical performance?*

   Yes, it promises to do the following:

   Increase nitrogen retention

   Increase $\dot{V}O_2$max (aerobic endurance)

   Increase strength

   Lower body fat

   Improve libido

2. *Does it contain a secret ingredient or formula?*

   There is no secret ingredient or formula; however, an online search reveals that 5-methyl-7-methoxy-isoflavone is a flavone that is part of the family of flavonoids.

3. *Can you recognize the ingredients or easily learn what they are intended for in the physical body?*

Flavonoids are associated with increased antioxidant capacity. It is known that any increase in the blood's antioxidant capacity after the consumption of flavonoid-rich foods is not caused directly by the flavonoids themselves but most likely by the increased uric acid levels that result from the metabolism of flavonoids. Scientists are now capable of tracing flavonoids' activity, and when large increases occur, the body actually looks to remove them.

4. *Is there only anecdotal evidence or testimonials to support the claims made regarding improvements in health or physical performance?*

   Yes, there is only anecdotal evidence regarding the efficacy of this supplement (despite the seller's claims there are dozens of studies to back the formulation). There is not a well-published paper in a scientific journal that supports it.

5. *Are the claims supported by substantial research indicating improvements in health or physical performance?*

   No, they are not.

6. *Who is advertising or selling the product? Celebrities? Star athletes? The person who invented the product?*

   There does not seem to be any one person behind the product, and really it is only the company that makes it that is promoting the product.

7. *Does the product potentially exaggerate that a nutrient frequently found in foods can significantly enhance performance?*

   Yes, and there is nothing to back up the claims.

8. *What is the cost of the supplement in relation to obtaining the same nutrient from foods?*

   The supplement is at least $60 for a one-month supply. Since higher levels of flavonoids do not appear to be beneficial, as long as adequate amounts are consumed in the form of foods, then this is an expense that is unnecessary. When you consider that the body actually looks to get rid of flavonoids when taken in too high a dose, the $60 spent really is a waste.

9. *Do the benefits sound too good to be true?*

   Yes!

Iron

Iron is the mineral that the body is most dependent on for creating a training adaptation. It is stored as ferritin in the body's bone marrow and is responsible for several important roles related to athletic training and performance. Iron is needed for making hemoglobin and myoglobin, the oxygen transporters of the body. It also helps with daily functions of other tissues in the body and, most important, aids in the use of fat as a fuel at rest and during exercise. Some athletes, especially females, are at risk for deficiencies because of iron lost in sweat, an increase in red blood cell breakdown, and loss of iron from bleeding in the GI tract and menses.

Iron is found in food sources that contain both heme and nonheme iron. Food sources with heme iron include meat, poultry, and fish. This type of iron is not affected by other foods in a meal and is best for ensuring a good iron status. Nonheme iron is the form found in vegetables, legumes, cereals, and other sources of grain. Its absorption can be enhanced by vitamin C, but it is also inhibited by calcium, tannic acid (found in tea), phytic acid (found in grains), and bran. As a result, only 3 to 8 percent of the iron found in these foods can be absorbed, so a far greater volume of food is required to achieve the intake of iron needed by the body. The recommended dietary allowance (RDA) is 8 mg for men and nonmenstruating women and 18 mg for women in their menstruating years. For adolescents, it is recommended that boys consume 11 mg and girls 15 mg per day. The amount of iron loss per day for these groups is 1.0 for men and nonmenstruating women, 1.4 up to 2.2 for menstruating women, 1.2 for boys, and 1.7 for girls. Iron requirements for men, women, and pregnant and lactating women are shown in table 8.1. The RDA takes into account the estimated losses a nonathletic person would have in a day in addition to the amount of iron that can be absorbed by the body. The amount of iron absorbed by the body is rarely past 10 percent of that which is available in consumed foods or supplements. Although iron absorption is slightly greater in people who are deficient, the overall absorption for these people rarely goes above 20 percent.

Iron deficiency can have a significant impact on an athlete's ability to gain benefits from training and eventually on work capacity and endurance. There are three stages of iron deficiency: depletion, iron-deficient erythropoiesis, and iron-deficiency anemia. The first stage of iron deficiency develops when the body's stores become depleted, indicated by a ferritin concentration of 12 micrograms per liter or less. As iron stores are depleted, the body increases absorption; however, if a person continues to consume less than they are losing, the second stage of iron deficiency begins. This is characterized by a decrease in blood iron levels and a significant decrease in the saturation of transferrin, the protein that transports iron in the blood. Transferrin receptor, a protein that takes up iron to the body's tissues, will increase. The third stage of iron deficiency results in a decreased hemoglobin concentration of less than 12 grams per deciliter for women and 13 grams per deciliter for men.

Recovery from the different stages of iron deficiency is dependent on the amount of heme iron sources incorporated into the diet, tolerance to iron supplementation, and the person's compliance. On average, it takes approximately 4 to 6 weeks to recover from the first stage of iron deficiency, 6 to 12 weeks for the second stage, and greater than 12 weeks for the third stage. The amount of iron necessary for athletes has been suggested to be higher than the RDA (as much as 50 percent) but has not been determined. Iron deficiency is high in certain athlete populations; thus, a proactive and preventative approach to ensuring iron status remains healthy is important. This can best be done by making heme iron part of the daily diet and through taking a multivitamin or iron supplement that contains up to the RDA.

Should iron deficiency be determined, supplementation with ferrous sulfate or ferrochel (iron bisglycinate) is an option. The dosage and frequency of iron supplemen-

Table 8.1   **Iron Requirements**

Age	Males	Females	Pregnancy	Lactation
9-13 years	8	8	n/a	n/a
14-18 years	11	15	27	10
19-50 years	8	18	27	9
51+ years	8	8	n/a	n/a

All values are in milligrams per day.

tation recommended by the Centers for Disease Control is up to 60 mg of elemental iron a day divided over three doses. Should an athlete experience the second or third stage of iron deficiency, a more aggressive approach under the supervision of a physician may be needed. If iron supplementation causes GI distress, the athlete should take the supplement every third day instead of daily. Iron status should always be checked after four to six weeks of supplementation; this will ensure that toxicity does not occur and that sufficient progress is being made by the athlete.

Calcium

Calcium is a mineral that assists in metabolism and is needed for optimal skeletal muscle function and bone formation. The majority of calcium should come from the intake of dairy products because these sources are highly bioavailable. Athletes consuming at least three servings of dairy per day will obtain at least 75 percent of the recommended dietary intake. When the caloric density of the diet is sufficient, athletes should be able to obtain the remaining calcium from other nondairy food sources. Calcium is also readily available in calcium-fortified orange juice, fortified breads and cereals, dark green vegetables, and soy products.

Bone density is of primary concern for athletes, especially those with a high incidence of stress fractures. The majority of bone mass accrues by the age of 21 to 25 years and is a result of the density in dietary intake, calcium intake, physical activity, and hormone levels. Studies have reported that female athletes who appear to have inadequate diets may be at risk for low bone density and potentially osteoporosis. Supplementation with calcium has been suggested to be a key part of improving bone density; however, when bone density is sufficient, calcium does not appear to further improve bone mass or lessen the risk for stress fractures. For those athletes who may require calcium supplementation to improve bone density, building up to an intake of 1,500 mg daily, in doses of at least 500 mg at a time, is recommended. There are various forms of calcium, with the two most common being calcium citrate and calcium carbonate. Calcium citrate can be taken at any time, whereas calcium carbonate needs to be taken with meals to improve its absorption. People tolerate calcium supplementation in different ways, and thus the ability to increase from one dose of 500 mg up to three doses will vary.

Zinc

The trace mineral zinc is important because it facilitates immune function and repair of tissues and is involved in many aspects of metabolism and DNA repair and synthesis. Zinc is a mineral that can also be lost in sweat (along with iron), and as a result athletes need to ensure that they are meeting daily requirements. Foods that are the greatest source of zinc are meats, seafood, and poultry. Adequate dietary intake will ensure that RDA levels are met. For zinc, this is 15 mg per day for men and 12 mg for women.

Zinc is a supplement that athletes associate with preventing illness, and as a result they may consume it in excess. Caution must be taken with zinc supplements or lozenges because they have the potential to inhibit the absorption of iron and copper, two very important minerals for optimal body function. There is no substantial evidence that zinc supplementation can enhance performance when food intake is adequate; thus, supplementing the diet with more than the recommended dietary allowance is not recommended.

Antioxidants

Antioxidants offer protection to the body's cells from oxidative stress. During metabolism, oxygen is reduced to form water, but a small percentage, 4 to 5 percent, is not completely reduced. Oxygen intermediates—called reactive oxygen species (ROSs)—are formed, and some of these are free radicals. These free radicals contain an unpaired electron in the outer orbital, which makes them very unstable. ROSs are harmful to the body's cells, but the body is capable of neutralizing ROSs with internal and external antioxidants. Popular dietary antioxidants include vitamin C, vitamin E, carotenoids, polyphenols, alpha-lipoic acid, ubiquinones, flavonoids, glutathione, and coenzyme Q_{10}.

However, when the production of ROSs exceeds this antioxidant defense system, oxidative stress takes place and may reduce performance capacity. Because of the higher oxygen consumption of athletes, there is also an increase in ROS production, and although oxidative stress has been linked to disease states, the significance of exercise-induced oxidative stress on athletes is somewhat unknown.

Research indicates that athletes may require slightly higher amounts of antioxidants than the recommended levels for nonathletes to combat the effects of exercise-induced oxidative stress. Getting antioxidants through foods such as fruits, vegetables, and whole grains supplies other compounds that have physiological protective functions, and these antioxidants may interact with others through eating a variety of foods. Because of this, it is recommended that eating up to three times the normal recommended intake of antioxidant nutrients from food sources can elicit health benefits. Antioxidant consumption matching the recommended dietary intake will likely not provide protection against oxidative stress in athletes. However, the exact amount and combination of antioxidant supplements that will alter the pro- and antioxidant balance and reduce exercise-induced oxidative stress are unknown. At this time, dietary sources of antioxidants are preferred over single or combined antioxidant supplements because of the possible negative health outcomes associated with prolonged use of high-dose supplements. It is important to remember that when taken in excess (high doses from supplements), antioxidants can become prooxidants and contribute to greater oxidative stress in the body. Lower-dose dietary supplements that include a variety of antioxidants may be beneficial for athletes who have a difficult time meeting their antioxidant needs with food, but supplements should not be a replacement for antioxidant-rich food sources.

Glucosamine and Chondroitin

Glucosamine and chondroitin promote joint health in athletes. The compound glucosamine is made from glucose and glutamine. It is needed to produce a molecule used in the repair and formation of cartilage in the body. The production of glucosamine decreases with age, which is why many older athletes choose to supplement it. As a supplement, glucosamine is manufactured from chitin, a substance that is found in the shells of lobster, crab, and other sea animals. More times than not, glucosamine is combined in supplemental form with chondroitin sulfate, a substance that is naturally found in cartilage. The combination of both targets osteoarthritis, a condition in which the joints become stiff and lose their elasticity, resulting in damage and possibly decreased range of motion, pain, and future deterioration, and is thought to assist in repairing damaged cartilage and thus improve the function of the joints, most commonly in the knees.

This certainly sounds promising; however, there is no good evidence that glucosamine supplementation is beneficial for athletes because of a lack of scientific studies. Some studies in military personnel show promise, but performance was not measured. Athletes using this supplement have seen benefits as measured subjectively, although this is not the case for all athletes. There have not been any reports of adverse effects of using this supplement to date.

Omega-3 Fatty Acids

Omega-3 fatty acids show great promise as supplements for athletes. Blood tests confirm that when athletes are in a cycle of high training load, inflammation is increased. An increase in inflammation can lead to less blood flow delivery to and from muscles, which means fewer nutrients getting to the muscles and a decreased efficiency in transporting waste away from the muscles. Omega-3 fatty acids have a direct effect on the inflammatory response. The essential fatty acid omega-3 has many other important functions, such as decreasing risk for coronary artery disease and hypertension, improving insulin sensitivity for athletes with type 2 diabetes, lowering triglycerides, and raising HDL (good) cholesterol.

From a performance standpoint, there is support for supplementing with omega-3 fatty acids, with positive effects seen on enhancing stroke volume (the amount of blood pumped from one ventricle of the heart) and cardiac output (the total volume of blood being pumped by the heart). Both are important for increasing oxygen delivery to the heart so it does not have to work as hard. Additionally, vasodilation in contracting muscles is enhanced. This is thought to be due to the fact that omega-3 fatty acids can increase the production of nitric oxide. Because of their anti-inflammatory properties, omega-3 fatty acids have also been found to have a protective effect in suppressing exercise-induced bronchoconstriction in athletes.

Omega-3 fatty acids are found in foods such as fatty fish (salmon, mackerel), walnuts, and flax products but often in smaller and less clinically significant amounts than what is found in supplements. Normal dosing of these supplements ranges from 3 to 10 grams per day for cardioprotective benefits and 1 to 2 grams per day for those not needing higher doses for any cardiovascular issues.

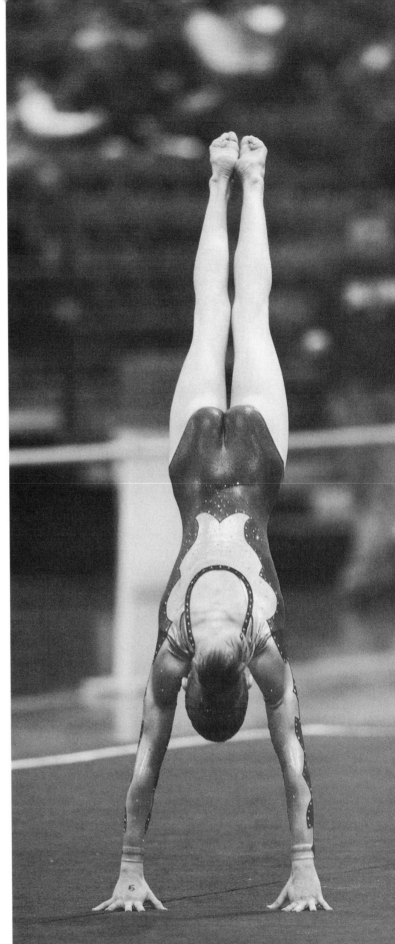

Athletes with low energy intakes, more common in aesthetic or weight class sports, may be at risk for B-vitamin deficiency.

B-Complex Vitamins

An adequate amount of B vitamins is needed for energy production and the building and repair of muscle tissue. The B vitamins thiamine, niacin, riboflavin, B_6, pantothenic acid, and biotin are involved in energy production during exercise, while folate and B_{12} are needed for the production of red blood cells, protein synthesis, and tissue repair.

For female and vegetarian athletes or those with disordered eating patterns, riboflavin, pyridoxine, folate, and B_{12} are frequently low. Although there has not been much research to support supplementation of B vitamins, some studies suggest that exercise may increase the need for these vitamins by as much as twice the normal recommended intake. Most recommendations are to eat more to acquire more of these vitamins, but this may not be realistic in some classes of athletes such as weight class, aesthetic, and some endurance, not to mention those with disordered eating. Clinically significant deficiencies of B vitamins can affect both health and performance, but marginal deficiencies of most of these vitamins have not been shown to have a negative effect on performance. However, the exceptions are severe deficiencies of B_{12}, folate, or both because this could increase the risk of anemia, which can have a direct negative impact on endurance performance.

Fiber

Fiber supplements can make fecal matter soft, which can benefit athletes who experience constipation. However, water intake must be increased or constipation can become worse. Some athletes will increase fiber in their diets too quickly, which can cause gas; thus, slowly increasing fiber-rich foods such as fruits, vegetables, and grains is recommended. Fiber-rich foods can also lead to a decrease in total cholesterol and low-density lipoproteins (LDLs) and are useful to include in an athlete's daily nutrition program if blood lipids are abnormal.

From a performance perspective, some athletes will significantly minimize the consumption of fiber-rich foods in the days leading up to competition as a method of reducing the chance of GI distress. The easiest way to do this is to use liquid meal supplements that are low in fiber. This fiber taper should be reversed after competition so that ill effects of a large amount of dietary fiber are not experienced.

Sport Supplements

Sport supplements can be used to enhance performance and adaptations in the nutrient timing windows before, during, and after training or competition. These supplements generally provide an additional or more convenient way to supply nutrients that can also be obtained from food. Supplements may provide carbohydrate, protein, fat, sodium, or fluid.

Postworkout Beverage

The main purpose of a postworkout beverage is to start the replenishment process of glycogen, fluid, and electrolytes and begin the body's adaptation process from the catabolic stresses of exercise. It is recommended that the postworkout beverage contain 1.0 to 1.2 grams of carbohydrate per kilogram of body weight, 10 to 25 grams of protein in the form of essential amino acids, at least 500 mg of sodium, and 24 ounces (720 ml) of fluid as a minimum depending on how much body weight is lost during the training session (table 8.2). These beverages should taste good and can be in either liquid or powder form. Liquids have the added benefit of improving

Table 8.2 **Recommended Composition of Postworkout and Preworkout Beverages**

Nutrient	Postworkout beverage	Preworkout beverage
Carbohydrate	1.0-1.2 g/kg of body weight	4-8 percent concentration
Protein	10-25 g	Up to 20 g
Sodium	Minimum 500 mg/L of fluid	110 mg per 8 oz (240 ml) of fluid
Fluid	24 oz/lb (1.6 L per kg) of body weight lost	.07-.10 oz/lb (4.7 to 6.6 ml/kg) of body weight 4 hours before .04-.10 oz/lb (2.7 to 6.6 ml/kg) of body weight 2 hours before

hydration status after a workout, but ingesting liquid versus solid sources is purely an individual choice. It may be beneficial for athletes who travel to use a powdered version, which is easier to travel with both nationally and internationally.

Preworkout Beverage

The main purpose of the preworkout beverage is to provide adequate fluid, carbohydrate, and sodium before competition. Therefore, this drink should contain between a 4 and 8 percent carbohydrate concentration and at least 110 mg of sodium per 8 ounces (240 ml) of fluid; fluid quantity should equal .07 to .10 ounces per pound (4.7 to 6.6 ml/kg) of body weight 4 hours before the workout and an additional .04 to .10 ounces per pound (2.7 to 6.6 ml/kg) of body weight 2 hours before (table 8.2). Some athletes, particularly those participating in strength training, may benefit from adding up to 20 grams of protein, specifically essential amino acids, to a carbohydrate beverage before training in an effort to maintain net protein synthesis rates and decrease the catabolic response of resistance training. It is important to note that most high-quality proteins are 40 percent essential amino acids by content.

During-Workout Beverage

The composition of a beverage consumed during a workout will depend greatly on the athlete, sport, intensity of training, and environmental conditions. It is generally recommended that athletes choose a beverage that contains between 4 and 8 percent carbohydrate and 500 to 700 mg of sodium per liter for training sessions lasting longer than an hour. The quantity will vary significantly because of individual differences. The forms of workout beverages, quantities, and ingredients vary as athletes determine their specific needs relative to their sports. In most weight-class sports where dehydrating to make weight is popular before a competition, the athletes rarely drink beverages during a workout because they do not want anything in their stomachs during physical contact with another competitor.

Electrolytes

Most athletes, depending on the sport, time of competition year, and sweat rate, will require more electrolytes than the recommended ranges. The main electrolytes found in sweat are sodium, chloride, potassium, calcium, and magnesium, and these are often the center of attention in supplementation. Depending on the sport and environmental conditions, sweat rates for athletes can range from .3 to 2.4 liters per hour. Sodium is the predominant electrolyte lost in sweat, and although there is a very wide range of sweat sodium loss during exercise, 1 gram of sodium per liter of fluid lost is the average.

There is no concrete recommendation regarding electrolyte intake before exercise, although many athletes consume salty foods and drinks beforehand to prevent hyponatremia. Consuming an adequate amount of salt on a daily basis, especially for salty sweaters, is recommended, and in some cases, salt tablets may be warranted during exercise as long as they are consumed with enough fluid to maintain fluid–electrolyte balance. Athletes should limit fluid intake to only what is needed to minimize dehydration and consume sodium-rich foods and beverages during exercise longer than 2 hours to prevent excessive drinking and thus risk of hyponatremia. It is currently recommended that athletes consume drinks containing 500 to 700 mg of sodium per liter; however, for many athletes who are salty sweaters, this may be too low. Athletes may experience fewer symptoms of hyponatremia and cramping when a higher amount of sodium is consumed.

Whey and Casein Protein

Both whey and casein protein are found in milk. Whey protein, found in very small amounts in milk (20 percent), is a by-product of cheese and curd manufacturing, while casein is responsible for making the curds. Whey protein has a higher-quality rating and is a complete protein containing all the essential amino acids. It is also rich in vitamins and minerals and has the highest branched-chain amino acid (leucine, isoleucine, and valine) content, which is important to athletes as described in chapter 4. Additionally, whey protein is a fast protein, meaning it is quick to enter the body to provide the essential amino acids and thus has a significant impact on protein synthesis. Because of this, most athletes will take whey protein immediately before and after exercise.

Casein protein is the predominant protein (80 percent) found in milk and has a good amino acid profile, but in contrast to whey, casein is considered a slow protein. It causes a more steady release of amino acids over a 3- to 4-hour period of time. Casein is not known to have a large impact on protein synthesis, but rather is known to suppress protein breakdown. The ideal scenario for athletes is to increase protein synthesis rates and decrease protein breakdown rates; using both whey and casein protein at different times throughout the day corresponding to workouts is therefore ideal. It is generally recommended that whey protein be used in the morning, before and after training, while casein is used in between meals and before bed if a protein snack is eaten.

Soy Protein

Soy protein does not contain as high a level of branched-chain amino acids as whey and casein protein but still contains all the essential amino acids. It is the protein found in soybeans, and some athletes will use soy as a vegetable option of protein since whey and casein come from animal products. Soy has beneficial health effects such as improving cardiovascular status and preventing obesity, and it is a complete protein source for vegetarian athletes.

Although soy protein also contains antioxidants that promote cardiovascular health and it has been shown that consuming soy protein in conjunction with strength training may promote muscle mass gains, milk proteins consumed after strength training may promote more rapid gains in muscle mass.

Ergogenic Aids

An ergogenic aid is a nutritional, physical, mechanical, psychological, or pharmacological intervention that can improve physical work capacity. Ergogenic aids typically work by acting on the central or peripheral nervous system to increase the storage or availability of a limiting substrate, provide a fuel source, reduce or neutralize by-products of metabolism, or facilitate recovery from training or competition. A number of products have been developed over the years and marketed as ergogenic aids; however, only a few have proven to be safe and of true benefit to performance.

Ergogenic aids are typically the most confusing class of supplement in athletics. Because they are not included in the nutrients that sustain life (carbohydrate, protein, fat, water, vitamins, minerals), they are typically thought of only as performance enhancing and for specific use pertaining to sport and not health. Ergogenic aids are not a form of nutrient and are not intended to replace good nutrition habits or training. They are intended for use at appropriate time points in an athlete's career, under the guidance of a physiologist, strength and conditioning coach, or nutritionist who can ensure they are used appropriately. The timing and dosage of some of the ergogenic aids are critical to ensure that side effects do not interfere with training or performance. Although we provide content on ergogenic aids, we do not necessarily endorse their use. Please be advised that the abuse or misuse of these ergogenic aids has potentially adverse side effects. Athletes should use ergogenic aids at their own risk under the close supervision of a qualified health professional.

Caffeine

Caffeine is considered a stimulant that directly affects the central nervous system. It has been shown to enhance endurance performance, reaction time, mental alertness, and cognitive function. Improvements in performance are thought to be a result of increased motor unit recruitment; by increasing the number of muscle crossbridges that can be formed, an athlete can generate more force production and thus power. A second means of performance improvement may be an increase in the number of beta-endorphins, which allows athletes to sustain a higher-quality performance for a longer period of time; thus, caffeine is acting centrally in the brain rather than locally at the muscle. Lastly, caffeine has also been shown to increase fat and carbohydrate oxidation, which can help supply energy to the working musculature at a faster rate.

The timing of caffeine ingestion is important to optimize its effects. In events of shorter duration, consuming a dose of .2 to .3 mg of caffeine per kilogram of body weight is recommended in the hour to 30 minutes before competition. In endurance events such as a marathon, a triathlon, or an ultraendurance competition, athletes tend to consume this dose 30 minutes before the start of the race and then continue to take in up to 20 mg of caffeine at 45-minute intervals. Caffeine is commonly taken in through gels, flat soda, coffee, and energy drinks as well as directly in pill or powder form as caffeine anhydrous, all of which can easily be purchased at a local drug store. Potential side effects of caffeine include dizziness, irritability, nausea, and nervousness.

Creatine

Creatine is a natural energy source that can be found in meat and fish. These animal sources of protein have anywhere between 3 and 7 grams of creatine per kilogram of body weight. Creatine supplementation has been shown to enhance performance in short maximal bouts and in events that require repeated bursts of powerful movements, such as tennis, soccer, field hockey, and football. It has also been shown to improve gains in muscle mass and improve the gains in muscle strength and power that can be obtained from resistance training.

The performance gains from creatine supplementation are thought to result from an improved ability to generate ATP through the ATP–CP energy system. By increasing the availability of creatine, ATP in the muscle cell can regenerate faster, improving energy supply and the ability to recover. As a result, muscle contraction at high force outputs can be maintained, and this is beneficial for training (especially if volume is high) and in competition where repeated explosive bursts are required. Creatine predominantly works by increasing work capacity and thus can create a training adaptation and improve the potential to increase muscle mass. The increase in work capacity allows the athlete to train harder and longer, and as a result the athlete obtains a higher level of power endurance.

Creatine supplementation can be done in several different ways. The traditional method is to have an initial loading phase in which 15 to 20 grams is consumed per day for five to seven days. After this period, a maintenance dose of 3 to 5 grams per day is consumed during the training cycle. A second approach to consuming creatine is to skip the loading phase and consume 3 to 5 grams per day throughout the desired training cycle. Regardless of the supplementation approach, creatine should most likely be taken for anywhere between three to eight weeks and then be discontinued for at least four weeks before being consumed again. Chronic creatine supplementation may reduce its effects, and thus cycling creatine may be necessary to continue receiving the desired benefits.

Several types of creatine are available on the market. Creatine monohydrate is the most common form sold; however, creatine salts, such as creatine citrate or pyruvate, are also available. No form of creatine is superior to another. All should have the same effect as long as they are of a pure quality. Potential side effects of creatine include allergic reactions and decreased urine output.

The timing of creatine consumption can also affect how well it is taken up by the muscle and retained. When creatine is consumed in the 30 minutes before exercise, it has been shown to stimulate uptake by the muscle for immediate use as a fuel source. Ingesting creatine immediately after exercise with a carbohydrate and protein beverage has been shown to facilitate retention of creatine in the muscle. Depending on the goal, creatine consumption may be divided into two doses, one that is consumed immediately before and the other immediately after training.

Sodium Bicarbonate

Sodium bicarbonate is considered to be a buffering compound that helps the body tolerate high levels of lactate. Buffers are considered beneficial in sports where anaerobic metabolism will predominate; thus, events lasting up to approximately 5 minutes in duration would potentially receive the greatest benefit. Reliance on anaerobic metabolism results in high levels of lactate, which will eventually hinder the ability to form muscle crossbridges and thus limit performance. Sodium bicarbonate helps buffer lactic acid, and as a result, hydrogen ions that would hinder muscle crossbridge formation are not able to do so; the muscle can consequently sustain a higher level of force production and thus more power.

More recent research has examined the effects of bicarbonate use during prolonged endurance events. This research indicates that events where aerobic metabolism predominates can also benefit. Benefits potentially include the ability to tolerate higher levels of lactic acid for a more prolonged period of time and a reduction in breathing rate, which would significantly help an athlete from a psychological standpoint. The sodium that is available may also be a key factor in improving performance. Sodium helps retain fluid in the body and as a result will increase blood volume. An increase in blood volume would then result in a more efficient heart rate response as well as an improved oxygen delivery and carbon dioxide removal system. There is still much to be learned about the potential benefits that bicarbonate can have on endurance performance.

The timing of sodium bicarbonate loading is necessary to obtain the maximal benefits it is capable of providing. There is an acute and long-term approach to loading. The acute method requires that athletes consume approximately .3 to .4 grams of bicarbonate per kilogram of body weight, starting 90 minutes to 3 hours before training or competition, while also consuming at least 16 ounces (480 to 600 ml) of a carbohydrate–electrolyte beverage. The long-term approach to loading allows the body to store bicarbonate over a six-day period. For long-term loading, .5 mg of bicarbonate per kilogram of body weight is consumed every 3 to 4 hours for six days before competition. Neither loading method appears to provide better results than the other; however, the long-term approach may be easier to maintain when athletes must compete for several days in a row and need to continue supplementing for performance purposes. Athletes competing in multiple-day events should continue with the recommended dosage all the way through the competition.

Determining the best means of consuming sodium bicarbonate is one of the most critical aspects of its use. Consumed in its raw form, sodium bicarbonate can lead to severe gastrointestinal side effects. Athletes can avoid these potential side effects in three ways: (1) Use no more than the recommended dose needed to achieve the desired effects, (2) utilize a milder form known as sodium citrate, and (3) consume the bicarbonate in gelatin capsules with a light carbohydrate–electrolyte solution (>6 percent).

The recommended doses for bicarbonate use were developed on athletes who weighed approximately 110 to 176 pounds (50 to 80 kg); thus, for athletes who weigh more or less, the dose may not be appropriate. When experimenting with bicarbonate, it is recommended that athletes begin with 50 percent of the suggested dose and then steadily increase in 25 percent increments to 100 percent. This should help prevent any of the unpleasant side effects that may come as a result of supplementation and will help the athletes further define their own tolerable ranges. Potential side effects of sodium bicarbonate supplementation include nausea, vomiting, diarrhea, headache, muscle pain, dry mouth, increased urination, decreased appetite, and constipation.

Beta-Alanine

Beta-alanine is an amino acid that is important for increasing carnosine concentrations in muscle. Carnosine is a peptide, and increased levels in the muscle can help buffer lactate and improve muscle function and thus muscle crossbridge formation. Recent studies show that supplementation with beta-alanine can result in increased muscle carnosine concentrations and improved performance. Supplementation at 40 to 65 mg/kg of body weight has been shown to delay fatigue, improve anaerobic and aerobic power production, and improve time to exhaustion, all of which indicate that beta-alanine can improve work capacity. In addition, one study found that combining beta-alanine with creatine resulted in greater strength gains and improvements in body composition than supplementing with creatine alone. Beta-alanine should be ingested throughout the day in doses equal to no more than 800 mg at any one point in time. Potential side effects when taken in large doses include flushing and tingling. Although it is a relatively new supplement, beta-alanine appears to be very promising as an ergogenic aid.

Glycerol

Glycerol is a lipid that is metabolized like carbohydrate. It traditionally is known as the backbone of a triglyceride because it holds the free fatty acids. Glycerol can also attract large amounts of water, and thus it may be used to hyperhydrate athletes who are in need of a greater total water capacity during competition. Traditionally, athletes use glycerol when competing in hot environments; however, athletes who are heavy sweaters regardless of the environment may find it of benefit. Recent research suggests that the addition of creatine to a glycerol solution can increase fluid retention and help to further regulate body temperature by increasing total body water. Increases in total body water help act as a "heat sink," and thus core body temperature will not rise as quickly.

Glycerol must be consumed in a slow and steady manner when the athlete is in a hydrated state. Possible side effects of glycerol consumption include headaches, nausea, and blurred vision. However, research has shown that the addition of creatine has the added benefit of eliminating side effects, most likely because it enables creatine to cross the blood–brain barrier and maintain fluid homeostasis, which prevents the fluid imbalance that can cause headaches. Glycerol can be consumed at a rate of 1 to 2 g/kg of body weight; higher doses can produce more significant side effects.

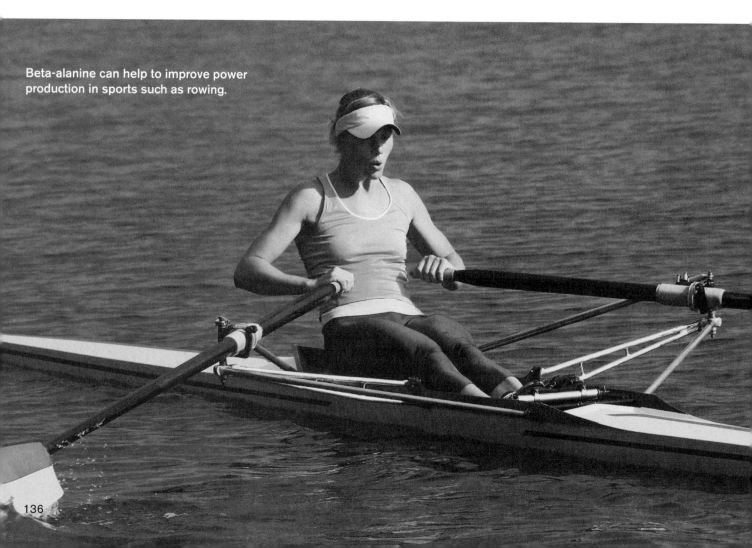

Beta-alanine can help to improve power production in sports such as rowing.

Beta-Alanine for Anaerobic Capacity

A heavyweight rower who was looking to improve her anaerobic capacity struggled to do so just through training. She had a very low maximal lactate level (7.2 mmol/L) in comparison to her teammates. Despite working hard to improve, the desired increases in power production and maximal lactate tolerance were not coming at the rate hoped for by the athlete and coach. Since this athlete's nutrition was already very well rounded, the next step was to look at ergogenic aids. For 10 weeks the athlete supplemented with increasing doses of beta-alanine. She started with 800 mg and continued to increase the dose every week by 800 mg until she reached almost 5,000 mg, which is the maximal dose (~65 mg/kg of body weight) recommended for her body weight of 165 pounds (75 kg). Every week the athlete's progress was monitored during her most demanding anaerobic interval training set. Over the 10-week period, she was able to increase power output significantly and increased the ability to tolerate lactic acid, as indicated by a maximal lactate of 9.6 mmol/L.

Loading with glycerol before a competition is one method of taking this supplement. Athletes consume the glycerol after the evening meal for the five nights before competition. It is recommended that the glycerol dose be divided into two liters of warm water, with 11 grams of creatine per liter of fluid and 40 grams of carbohydrate–electrolyte solution.

Glycerol can also be consumed on the day of competition and in competition. In the 2.5 hours before the event, athletes can do the following: Using a 20 percent glycerol solution, drink 5 milliliters per kilogram (ml/kg) of body weight. At 30 and 45 minutes after this time point, consume water at the rate of 5 ml/kg of body weight. At 60 minutes, consume more of the glycerol solution at 1 ml/kg of body weight along with 5 ml/kg of water. At 90 minutes, another 5 ml/kg of water should be consumed. This should leave approximately an hour before any exercise is to be started. For events lasting longer than 2 hours, consuming a 5 percent glycerol solution at a rate of 15 to 30 fluid ounces (450 to 900 ml) per hour may also be beneficial. Most athletes do not like this method because there is a feeling of discomfort in the gut as the glycerol is absorbed, and psychologically this may be detrimental. Athletes tend to prefer loading in the days leading up to the race.

Phosphagen

Supplementation with phosphagen has been shown to improve power output, improve oxygen extraction, and improve exercise capacity by reducing lactate values at submaximal workloads and increasing the ability to tolerate lactate during maximal efforts. The benefits are potentially related to the timing of phosphagen ingestion. When phosphagen is consumed at 4 grams per day over a three- to six-day period, it appears to improve performance; however, the benefits may depend on the timing of the last dose, which needs to be consumed 2 to 3 hours before the exercise bout. However, not all studies examining phosphagen supplementation have shown this. Only those athletes who have tested performance within a few hours after the last dose have shown improvements. Regardless, it appears that phosphagen consumed several hours before exercise can improve performance.

Colostrum (Bovine)

Colostrum is the first milk secreted by animals after giving birth. It is a rich source of growth factors, immunoglobulins, and antimicrobial proteins and also provides protein, carbohydrate, vitamins, and minerals. As a result, colostrum is thought to have the potential to improve the immune system, enhance recovery from exercise, and promote muscle growth. Supplementation with 50 to 60 grams of colostrum per day has led to significant improvements in anaerobic performance, ability to perform a second bout of training, and markers of immune function. These improvements have not been observed in all studies examining performance and health status; however, the colostrum dose in these studies was only 20 grams per day, which could explain the differences found. At present, it appears this supplement can potentially benefit athletes in the areas of immune and muscle function.

Beta-Hydroxy-Beta-Methylbutyrate (HMB)

HMB is a metabolite that comes from the branched-chain amino acid leucine. It is thought to be a rate-limiting factor in muscle building. It has been suggested that HMB works by enhancing the ability of leucine to inhibit muscle breakdown. Studies indicate that supplementation with HMB at 1.5 to 3.0 grams per day may result in greater gains in muscle mass as a result of resistance training, especially in athletes who are just beginning a resistance training program. As a result, some studies also show increased power output, and thus the maximal capacity to do work is improved. However, not all studies have shown these improvements with supplementation, and when used in conjunction with creatine or essential amino acids, there does not appear to be an additional benefit of using HMB with these already anabolic supplements.

Amino Acids

Amino acids are the building blocks of protein. Studies indicate that essential amino acids (EAAs) and the nonessential amino acids glutamine and tyrosine may be the most beneficial to consider for supplementation. Essential amino acids promote amino acid uptake by the muscles and muscle synthesis, facilitate creatine uptake by the muscles, and improve glycogen storage by enhancing insulin's response to carbohydrate. All of these help minimize muscle damage that may occur as a result of training, improve recovery from exercise, and enhance body composition. The minimal dose necessary appears to be 6 grams of EAAs. The time points that show the greatest benefit are 30 minutes before resistance training and within 45 minutes after cardiovascular and resistance training. Continuing to ingest EAA at 1 and 2 hours after training also appears to be of benefit. This would help maximize muscle synthesis and glycogen restoration.

Tyrosine, a nonessential amino acid, has shown the greatest promise for events that require prolonged or high levels of concentration or that require a stable mood and the control of physical stress, such as prolonged endurance events and technical sports such as golf, shooting, and archery, all of which have the potential to produce mental fatigue. The effects of tyrosine supplementation on performance are debatable. Although studies have not always noted significant improvements via statistics, an improvement in cycling time-trial performance of 1 to 2 minutes is significant to an athlete. The studies also reported a decreased rating of perceived effort.

Two grams of tyrosine 30 to 60 minutes before exercise has been shown to enhance performance. In addition, consuming tyrosine throughout the day also appears to offer performance benefits, which is critical for athletes competing in multiple rounds that span across the day. The suggested total daily dose of tyrosine ranges anywhere between 25 and 150 mg/kg of body weight, with 100 mg/kg reported as the average dose. For most athletes, this puts the dose at approximately 3 to 12 grams per day, and spreading it over three or more time points is recommended.

Glutamine is the amino acid used by cells of the immune system. It is made in muscle and is the most abundant amino acid in the body. Glutamine decreases after intense exercise and remains lowered until the body recovers. Studies show a relationship between glutamine status and athletes who may be overtrained. In a fatigued state, such as that experienced by an overtrained athlete, glutamine can become depressed and possibly make the body more susceptible to illness. In a state of overtraining, athletes are considered to be chronically underrecovered, which may explain the lowered blood glutamine levels reported in these athletes. This is usually a result of undereating for the energy expended because appetite is often suppressed in overtrained athletes. Glutamine supplementation at .9 mg/kg of body weight may help protect the function of immune system cells, thus lowering the potential for illness. Some researchers also suggest that glutamine supplementation during periods of intense training may keep athletes from becoming overtrained; however, more research is needed in this area.

Conclusion

Dietary and sport supplements as well as ergogenic aids have the potential to complement an athlete's nutrition plan when they are used appropriately. In today's competitive world, more and more athletes are participating in high-level sport at the amateur and professional levels. In addition, an even greater number of people are competing as recreational athletes and seeking to achieve the best results they can possibly obtain. Although many supplements have been shown to be beneficial to sport performance, it is critical that athletes first and foremost ensure a good nutrition plan before trying these products.

Nutrient Timing in Changing Environments

The body is constantly adapting to its external environment so that homeostasis can be maintained. When a person is stressed by environmental changes, the brain immediately initiates an adaptive response to minimize strain and reestablish balance in the body's systems. The goal of this chapter is to describe acclimatization to altitude, heat, and cold, as well as changes in air quality. It also describes the changes in fuel use at rest and in training and how timing nutrient ingestion becomes even more critical for improving the body's function in these environments.

Altitude

Altitude is the environment that results in a reduced air pressure, and thus a lower amount of oxygen is available with every breath a person takes. This causes **hypoxia,** a state where the rate of oxygen supply cannot meet the oxygen used by the body's cells. As a result, energy requirements from aerobic metabolism—which is dependent on oxygen—decrease, and an increase in energy from anaerobic metabolism is required to sustain energy needed by the body, especially when performing any type of work. Athletes train at a variety of different altitudes, and mountaineers on expedition often climb in high altitudes. Moderate altitude can be defined as anywhere between 4,900 and 9,800 feet (1,500 and 3,000 m), high altitude as 9,800 feet to 18,000 feet (3,000 to 5,500 m), and very high altitude as anything above 18,800 feet (5,500 m). In this chapter, we focus on needs at moderate altitude, as these are most relevant to the athletic population.

Training at altitude can bring about improvements in the number of **red blood cells** available to transport oxygen. It can also increase the body's ability to utilize fat as a fuel source and improve the ability to buffer lactic acid. Together, these can result in an improved exercise economy and an enhanced ability to recover when training and competing at sea level.

hypoxia – A state where the rate of oxygen supply cannot meet oxygen utilization by the cells of the body.

red blood cell – The cell that is the principal means of delivering oxygen throughout the body. Red blood cells contain hemoglobin, which is responsible for binding oxygen.

Initial adaptation to altitude (figure 9.1) is a result of an increase in breathing and heart rate to supply oxygen to the body's tissues. On the first day of altitude exposure, the long-term adaptation to altitude is initiated through an increase in production of erythropoietin (EPO), the hormone responsible for the stimulation of new red blood cells. Over a 30-day period, this hormone helps facilitate an increase in red blood cells that can result in an increased ability to transport oxygen. This process is highly dependent on iron to form the red blood cells; however, altitude can also result in altered nutrient absorption, and thus it is important to ensure iron's availability so the desired training adaptation can be obtained.

Altitude also increases fluid loss because of water lost through the lungs and an increased frequency of urination. Together, these factors can have a significant impact on an athlete's ability to train and obtain the adaptations from altitude that are so beneficial to performance. Each of these factors is explained along with strategies designed to overcome these challenges at altitude.

Energy Needs

When athletes journey to altitude, it is not uncommon for them to lose body weight if they are not cautious about their food and fluid intake. In males, up to 6.6 pounds (3 kg) of weight loss has been reported. This can be attributed to the initial increase in resting metabolic rate (RMR), alterations in nutrient absorption, an increase in

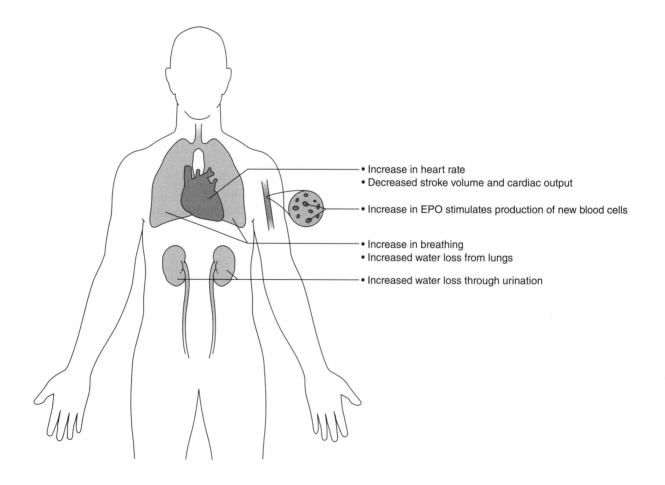

- Increase in heart rate
- Decreased stroke volume and cardiac output

- Increase in EPO stimulates production of new blood cells

- Increase in breathing
- Increased water loss from lungs

- Increased water loss through urination

Figure 9.1 Adaptations occurring as a result of altitude exposure.

relative exercise intensity, and increased fluid loss; in addition, appetite can be inhibited, resulting in even further losses in body weight. The increase in RMR has been reported as anywhere between 7 and 14 percent higher than at sea level during the first week of **acclimatization** and is dependent on how dramatically altitude affects a person. This is attributed to an increased need for energy at rest and the increased energy spent in training. As an athlete acclimatizes to altitude, RMR is reduced back to sea-level values as the body improves its ability to deliver oxygen and derive energy from fat stores.

At approximately 4,900 feet (1,500 m) of altitude is where most athletes begin to experience a decline in their aerobic energy system. Athletes rely heavily on anaerobic metabolism during the first 10 days of the altitude acclimatization period, regardless of the exercise intensity. At this altitude, decrements in aerobic work capacity are about 3 percent in comparison to sea level, and for every 90 feet (300 m) above this point, it can be assumed that work capacity will be reduced even further as a result of aerobic power being compromised by approximately another 3 percent. As a result, an athlete's ability to sustain high-intensity training is reduced, and recovery is impaired and takes longer to achieve. Despite acclimatization to altitude, an athlete's maximal work capacity will never be the same as that achievable at sea level, primarily because the body limits maximal cardiac output. Cardiac output is a function of heart rate and stroke volume (volume of blood ejected with every beat of the heart) and is thought to be reduced at altitude as a protective mechanism to ensure that the body's oxygen supply to the brain and other organs of the body is not compromised.

Since maximal work capacity is reduced, the same submaximal workload will be a higher relative percentage of maximal capacity and as a result will increase the energy needed to perform training (figure 9.2). A simple method of monitoring training during the acclimation period is to use blood lactate levels. Blood lactate levels during low-intensity aerobic training have been reported to be as high as 10 millimoles per liter (mmol/L) during the first days of altitude training and after a 10-day acclimation period have returned to approximately 1 to 2 mmol/L. This indicates the initial increased reliance on anaerobic metabolism and the shift that occurs back to the aerobic energy system.

Despite increases in energy expenditure when training at altitude, athletes do not appear to automatically increase caloric intake; nor has it been shown that people prefer an increase in one macronutrient over another. During the first week of acclimatization to altitude, the reliance on carbohydrate as a fuel source is greater because of the increased use of anaerobic metabolism for energy production at rest and in training. The choice of whether or not to focus on increasing carbohydrate content at altitude has always been heavily debated. Improvements in aerobic metabolism over three weeks of training at moderate and high altitudes are the result of an increased ability to utilize fat at rest and during exercise. Although there is initially a greater reliance on carbohydrate, the greatest benefits appear to come from matching the energy expended rather than relying on any one macronutrient to compensate for the increase in energy demands. Thus, setting a timeline that will allow for an increase in energy intake should help ensure that fuel needs are met.

relative exercise intensity – Defines exercise intensity based on a relative percentage of maximal workload achieved.

acclimatization – Adaptation (improved tolerance) to a chronic change in environment.

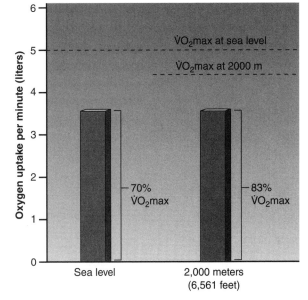

Figure 9.2 Because $\dot{V}O_2$max is reduced at altitude, an athlete working at a given intensity—here, running at a 6-minute-mile pace—is working at a higher percentage of maximal capacity. At sea level, this pace requires this athlete to work at only 70% of $\dot{V}O_2$max, but at 2,000 m, the same pace represents 83% of $\dot{V}O_2$max and requires more energy.

free radical – A molecule that can cause damage to the body because its charge is unbalanced.

Another critical reason for ensuring that energy demands are met is the immune system. Several responses associated with altitude training can compromise the body's immune function. Increased training stress along with the low-oxygen environment can lead to increased formation of **free radicals** in the body that can harm an athlete's tissues. This can tax the body's natural ability to fight off disease as antioxidants stored to help promote the immune system are reduced as a result of being utilized to decrease the number of free radicals in the body. In addition, athletes may experience an increase in the number of upper respiratory tract infections (URTIs) because the air at altitude is dryer than at sea level. Athletes are already prone to URTIs because of the large volume of air exchange they experience with training. Along with a negative energy balance, these factors can lead to an increased risk for illness, and as a result training can be compromised. The only macronutrient known to significantly protect the immune system during times of increased stress is carbohydrate, ideally from fruits that are rich in antioxidants. Thus, it may be optimal to increase carbohydrate intake through a variety of antioxidant-rich fruits to support and defend the immune system.

Frequency of eating is most likely the ideal way to ensure that energy needs are met at altitude. In previous chapters, we mention that eating approximately every 3 hours is necessary to maintain stable blood glucose levels. In the case of altitude exposure, eating every 2 hours is recommended, especially immediately before and after training sessions, to ensure fuel availability. Depending on the purpose of a training session, it may be necessary to focus on carbohydrate to ensure that quality can be maintained; however, if the training goal is to increase the ability of the body to use fat as a fuel source, just ensuring that energy is available will suffice. After the first week to 10 days of acclimatization, aerobic metabolism has returned, and the body has an increased ability to use fat as a fuel source; thus, at this point in time, the timing and source of fuel need to be matched to the desired training outcome, just as they would be at low altitude.

Iron

The trace mineral iron becomes even more important at altitude. The demand for iron is significantly greater, and the body's ability to absorb iron is improved. Before ascending to altitude, it is critical that athletes have adequate iron stores and not be in any stage of iron deficiency, as described in chapter 8. Iron must be available to help increase red blood cells by assisting in the formation of **hemoglobin** as well as myoglobin, the oxygen transporter of the muscle cell. Iron also helps to increase the activity of enzymes that are associated with fat metabolism.

hemoglobin – A molecule in red blood cells that is responsible for carrying oxygen throughout the body.

Should any form of iron deficiency exist, training adaptations that promote fat utilization during exercise and an improved economy will be lost. Training at altitude while in a state of iron deficiency is therefore not advised, and it is important to prevent a decline of iron stores. Studies examining iron supplementation in athletes training at altitude have found a more favorable iron and red blood cell status throughout the exposure. Athletes in an iron-sufficient state should consume the RDA (18 mg elemental iron for females; 8 mg elemental iron for males) as an insurance policy while training at altitude. This is recommended only as long as there is no danger of iron toxicity, as evidenced by ferritin stores no greater than 200 micrograms per liter for women and 300 for men and a transferrin saturation no greater than 45 percent.

Athletes who are going to train or exercise heavily at altitude may want to have their ferritin stores and other markers of iron status tested beforehand. If this is not possible, then taking the RDA in the form of ferrochel or ferrous sulfate for approximately a month before and during altitude training should help prevent iron deficiency.

Because only 2 to 8 mg (approximately 10 percent of ingested iron) is absorbed at any one time, it may be wise to split the RDA dose into three servings and take one-third of the dose at every meal.

A dose of iron greater than the RDA is not advised for several reasons. First, the intake of iron in large doses is a catalyst for creating free radicals and potentially causing damage to body tissues. Second, zinc and iron compete for absorption in the body. Large doses of iron have the potential to interfere with zinc absorption and as a result would interfere with the important roles that zinc plays in metabolism, muscle function and healing, bone formation, and DNA repair.

Fluid Loss

The ability to maintain a hydrated state in training is critical for optimal aerobic and anaerobic endurance, strength, and power. Hydration at altitude is even more critical because of the dry air; however, it is harder to achieve because most athletes already tend to voluntarily dehydrate, and the hormones that normally assist with fluid reabsorption in the kidneys and the body react to the reduced oxygen supply by increasing urine production. At altitude, the body naturally increases urination to rid the body of water in the blood so that the red blood cells become more concentrated and in turn improve oxygen delivery to the body's tissues. This occurs for as long as acclimatization to altitude is needed. It has been suggested that acclimation may take up to a year when living continuously at altitude, and with intermittent altitude exposure, full adaptation may never actually occur. In addition, the altitude environment may also be cold, which will increase urination even further. As a result of potentially cooler skin and body temperatures, athletes tend to increase restricted drinking and will not be stimulated to drink.

Significant fluid loss also occurs at altitude through the respiratory tract and skin. As a result of dry air conditions and an increase in breathing rate, the body loses a larger amount of fluid through the lungs at rest and especially during training. To ensure that an athlete drinks adequate fluids and does not compromise training, a timing system of frequent consumption of 2 to 4 ounces (60 to 120 ml) of fluid throughout the day is best. Fluid intake should match sweat losses and contain electrolytes in order to aid in fluid retention and replace electrolytes lost in sweat. This method will also help ensure that athletes are not consuming large volumes of fluid at any one time, which can lead to increased urination and create a vicious cycle of fluid intake and loss for an athlete that can be very discouraging.

Heat and Humidity

The body naturally produces heat at rest as a result of breaking down energy stores. During exercise the amount of heat produced is proportional to exercise intensity, and this raises a person's **core body temperature.** As the brain senses an increase in core temperature, blood flow is increased and taken away from the core of the body. This results in an enhanced cardiac output, which is evidenced by an increased heart rate at rest and during exercise. The blood is distributed to working muscles to facilitate their function by maintaining oxygen delivery and increasing the removal of waste and heat. Blood flow will also increase to the body's surface (skin), where heat is then removed through sweating.

The body uses four different methods—evaporation, convection, radiation, and conduction—to remove heat from the body so that severe **hyperthermia** (very high increases in body temperature) does not occur. Evaporation removes heat through

core body temperature – The temperature at which the internal organs and bodily systems function at an optimal level. It is considered a key aspect of the body's ability to control its operating temperature within a constant range.

hyperthermia – A condition in which the body is producing more heat than it can remove.

Nutrition to Support Altitude Training

A group of collegiate runners decided to try altitude training for eight weeks in the summer in an attempt to improve their endurance performance for the upcoming cross country season. They spoke to their coach about using a training plan that incorporated living and training at altitude. None of the athletes or the coach had ever been to altitude for training purposes. They went to a moderate altitude of 8,000 feet (2,450 m) with warm weather. Training went fine for the first five days. They experienced the usual increases in heart rate and breathing rate, but it was nothing the athletes thought was limiting them. Several days later, a couple of the athletes began to feel tired all throughout the day, and one member of the group had to stop training because of a severe headache and exhaustion. The remaining members of the group had to significantly slow their training pace.

A local professional runner saw the college students and asked how the trip was going. When he heard the issues, he contacted a local physiologist to ask for help. After reviewing their symptoms, the physiologist looked at the following items for each athlete: (1) iron status by assessing ferritin (iron stores), serum iron, and hemoglobin; (2) hydration status; and (3) the amount of carbohydrate and overall energy intake.

The athletes who were feeling tired showed low ferritin, serum iron, and hemoglobin levels indicating they had third-stage iron deficiency. All the other athletes had either stage-one or stage-two iron deficiency that was indicated by low ferritin, low serum iron, or both. All the athletes were significantly dehydrated, and the food they were taking in was not only missing the necessary carbohydrate but was also too low in energy intake for the volume of training they were attempting to do.

The athletes with second- and third-stage iron deficiency were advised to return home, and those with first-stage iron deficiency were placed on iron supplementation recommended by a local doctor. Those who remained at altitude took the next three days off from training to restore their bodies in terms of hydration and energy. Before they resumed training, they were shown how to match their fluid intake with sweat losses and rehydrate with fluids that contained electrolytes. They were also told to increase carbohydrate intake by consuming a carbohydrate snack before training and immediately after training. They also snacked more frequently throughout the day on light fruits to increase their carbohydrate intake, and they consumed meals that were high in complex carbohydrate and contained red meat at least three times per week.

sweating and is highly dependent on the amount of moisture in the air. In hot, dry conditions sweat is quickly dissipated; as the moisture content of air (i.e., humidity) increases, sweat cannot be readily removed, and less heat can be eliminated through this method. In a hot, dry environment evaporation accounts for up to 90 percent of heat loss. When humidity increases to greater than 50 percent, the body must increase reliance on other methods to remove heat. If this is not feasible, heat will continue to be stored by the body, and exercise intensity and duration will eventually be reduced.

The other means of removing heat is through nonevaporative methods that require an increase in heat loss to the environment or an object that is cooler than the body's temperature. In radiation, heat is given off by one object (the athlete) and is absorbed by the environment or another object that the person is in contact with (e.g., the ground). In convection, heat is lost by a person moving through a current (air or fluid). Conduction is the transfer of heat to another object through touch (e.g., the hand touching a cold surface) and in most situations accounts for very little heat loss.

When athletes move from a cool or moderate temperature to a hot environment, proper acclimatization to the heat over a two-week period before competing or training at full volume and intensity is probably the most important thing they can do. Athletes who experience hyperthermia when competing or training in the heat have usually not acclimatized appropriately. Acclimatization can be done by slowly increasing training volume and then intensity and by training at the coolest times of the day. The body's response to acclimatization is depicted in figure 9.3.

During the first five days of heat exposure, the adaptations of a decreased heart rate and perceived exertion to a training bout will occur. This is a result of an increase in plasma volume and the start of an increased retention of electrolytes (primarily sodium) in the sweat and urine. By day 10, core body temperature is decreased as the brain resets and increases sweat rate to compensate during exercise. The full increase in sweat rate is completed by day 14. Complete adaptation is also marked by a significant shift from anaerobic to aerobic metabolism and thus a greater reliance on fat as a fuel source rather than carbohydrate. The increased reliance on fat can be highly attributed to a reduction in strain on the body as a result of increased heat removal through a raised sweat rate, a decreased relative exercise intensity, and a decreased number of muscle fibers needed to perform the same amount of work. Together, these markers are evidence of a complete adaptation to the heat.

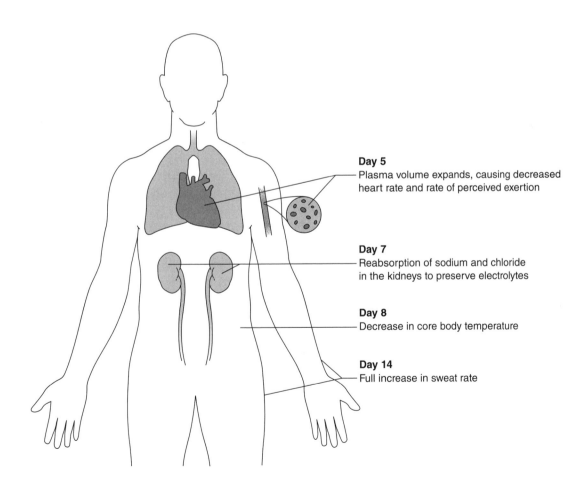

Day 5
Plasma volume expands, causing decreased heart rate and rate of perceived exertion

Day 7
Reabsorption of sodium and chloride in the kidneys to preserve electrolytes

Day 8
Decrease in core body temperature

Day 14
Full increase in sweat rate

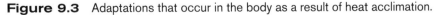

Figure 9.3 Adaptations that occur in the body as a result of heat acclimation.

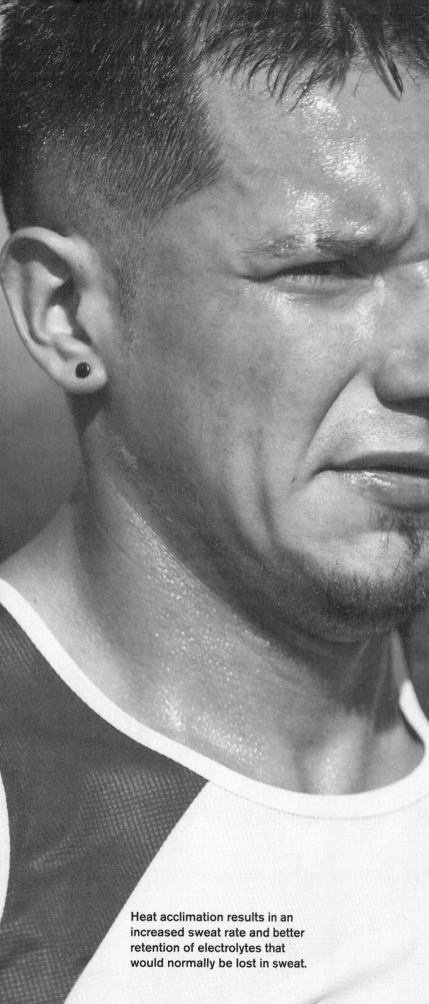

Heat acclimation results in an increased sweat rate and better retention of electrolytes that would normally be lost in sweat.

Energy and Hydration Needs

Ensuring that an athlete takes in adequate fuel and fluid during exercise in the heat is important to minimize injury and prevent premature fatigue. An athlete moving from a cool or moderate temperature to one that is hot experiences several shifts in metabolism that must be accounted for during training. At rest, RMR is decreased on average by approximately 5 percent. This is attributed to a decreased need to maintain body temperature because the environment helps do this; however, a hot environment can lead to decreased appetite, and as a result athletes need to be careful that they meet their energy needs.

Training in the heat increases demands on the body's metabolism in proportion to the increase in environmental heat. With a significant shift toward a more anaerobic metabolism, initial exposure results in increased carbohydrate use and decreased fat utilization; an increased sweat rate also leads to greater fluid losses. This happens because the athlete is working at a higher relative percentage of maximal capacity and because an increase in muscle temperature decreases muscle efficiency. When muscle temperature increases, muscle crossbridges fatigue at a higher rate; thus, the number of muscle fibers recruited over time will need to increase so that work capacity can be sustained. Depending on how well athletes acclimatize to a hot environment, they may or may not improve their reliance on fat as a fuel source. However, with heat acclimation, appropriate fueling and hydration strategies, and body-cooling techniques (e.g., cooling vest, cold showers or baths, hand and feet immersion in cool water, cool towels or ice packs), an athlete should be able to train and perform in such a harsh environment.

Because an athlete's body temperature is higher in warmer environments, the desire to eat can be significantly reduced; thus, it is important for an athlete to identify foods and fluids that taste pleasant at rest and during exercise. It is best to have a wide variety of palatable foods and fluids available and to make part of the recovery meal fluid based. Energy needs can be met through several different means. The types of fluid ingested and the amount of residue a food contains should be considered. The first strategy is to increase the calorie content of fluids used to rehydrate (e.g., meal replacements, carbohydrate–electrolyte beverages, juices, smoothies, iced tea). A second option is to increase low-residue foods eaten as snacks every 30 minutes to an hour in between meals. These foods are easier to digest and do not indicate to the receptors of the stomach that it is full. In addition, less heat is produced as these foods digest, and as a result, this will help control body temperature. Examples of high- and low-residue foods are listed in table 4.1 on page 73-74.

It is not uncommon for fluid loss to exceed the amount able to be taken in during training. Fluid ingestion can considerably improve the body's ability to minimize heat storage by helping to maintain sweat rate and providing a cooling sensation when ingesting fluids that are below body temperature. A timeline for fluid ingestion is important for coping with the heat. The timeline needs to ensure that an athlete enters each training session well hydrated and that hydration begins immediately after training and if possible is also incorporated into training. The temperature of a beverage can significantly influence how palatable it will be to an athlete and how quickly it can absorbed by the body. Cool fluids are best when training in a hot environment; when at rest, fluids that are at room temperature or slightly cooled will be better tolerated. The timeline shows guidelines for maintaining hydration when training in a hot environment.

Timeline

Hydration Guidelines for Hot Environments

- **Upon waking:** Consume 20 oz (600 ml) of fluid. Always ensure that half of the fluid volume contains electrolytes (milk, juice, smoothie, carbohydrate and protein meal replacement).
- **In the hour before training:** Consume 20 oz (600 ml) of fluid (if not right after waking).
- **During training:** If possible, consume 4 to 6 oz (120 to 180 ml) of fluid every 15 to 20 minutes.
- **Immediately after training:** Consume 20 oz (600 ml) of water or carbohydrate-electrolyte beverage.
- **After training:** Consume 4 to 8 oz (120 to 240 ml) of fluid every 15 to 20 minutes throughout the day until the amount of sweat lost from training is replaced. Multiple training sessions will most likely require that athletes drink continually throughout the day to keep up with fluid loss.
- **Before sleeping:** Consume 20 oz (600 ml) of fluid.

Hyperhydration

In athletes who have high sweat rates and whose fluid consumption and absorption cannot match sweat production, a hyperhydration strategy may be necessary for competition. Glycerol, the carbon backbone of a triglyceride, can aid in hyperhydration since it attracts water and can aid in the retention of fluids. In addition, recent research shows that the combination of glycerol with creatine can significantly increase the amount of water that can be held by the body. Creatine assists by drawing increased amounts of water into the muscle cell and thus acts as a "heat sink," keeping the body's core temperature reduced to prevent overheating. At the same time, blood flow can be maintained to a greater extent because of the increased pool of fluid throughout the body, thus allowing sweat rate to be maintained. Chapter 8 describes the best method for consuming a glycerol and creatine hyperhydration solution.

Heat Illness

When athletes do not appropriately manage heat removal from the body through increased fluid and electrolyte intake, heat illness can occur. The first level of heat illness is signaled by cramping in the working musculature, commonly termed *exercise-associated muscle cramps*. This is frequently a result of either low sodium levels in the body, significant dehydration, or both. It can easily be treated by ingestion of a rehydration solution that contains approximately one-third of a teaspoon of table salt per liter of fluid. This form of heat illness is usually caused by not being acclimatized to the heat.

The second degree of illness is heat exhaustion. This occurs in athletes who have very high sweat rates, are exerting themselves maximally, and have a significant mismatch between the amount of sweat produced to cool the body and the amount of fluid that can be taken in during training or competition. As a result of the significant dehydration and the inability to dissipate heat, these athletes also have a significantly elevated core body temperature (above 102 degrees Fahrenheit, or 39 degrees Celsius). If caught before they reach the point of heatstroke, these people will experience only mild symptoms of impaired mental function. They are not yet an extreme medical emergency and can be treated with rest, whole-body cooling, and replacement of fluids through oral rehydration or intravenous fluids.

When athletes continue exercising in the heat despite signs of intolerance and exhaustion, the third degree of heat illness may occur. Heatstroke is characterized by complete failure of the body to control temperature and is frequently associated with body temperatures greater than 104 degrees Fahrenheit (40 degrees Celsius). Dehydration is typically so severe that sweating will stop, and all the body's systems will stop functioning properly. This is attributed to a malfunctioning of the brain under such high temperatures, and as a result, nerve function and muscle control are lost. The damage that occurs both physically and mentally is dependent on the duration and intensity of the hyperthermia. This form of heat illness is best relieved through whole-body cooling via immersion in water (not ice) and must be treated by medical staff.

Overhydration and Hyponatremia

Hyponatremia is an abnormally low concentration of sodium in the blood. It is thought to be a result of large consumptions of water that is retained by the body, thus diluting the sodium in the blood; from sweat volume and sodium loss being so great that sodium is depleted in the body ("salty sweaters"); or a combination of both. Recent research suggests that the first scenario is most likely in recreational athletes, and in professional ultraendurance athletes, sodium loss is more likely the cause. Regardless of the cause, athletes must take measures to ensure that hyponatremia does not occur. For athletes who compete in events greater than 4 hours in duration, it is important that fluids contain electrolytes or that food or supplements with adequate salt (around 200 mg) are consumed throughout competition. At least 200 mg of sodium should accompany every 8 ounces (240 ml) of beverage consumed.

One strategy used by athletes who are salty sweaters is to increase sodium through diet in the weeks leading up to the race and in competition. Sodium balance in the body takes approximately 8 to 10 days to occur, and when done through increased salting of foods and ingesting foods with higher salt content, most athletes can adjust within this time frame and without complications. It is not recommended to consume a continuous high-sodium diet outside this time period for two primary reasons. The first is that high-sodium diets for long periods of time can be unhealthy and lead to increased risk of high blood pressure and heart disease. The second, and most important from a performance standpoint, is that chronic high-sodium loading will not provide an edge because the body would adapt and not be given the extra boost provided by short-term high-sodium consumption.

Cold Exposure

Athletes who train in cold environments must work at maintaining body temperature, not only by wearing clothing that keeps them well insulated but also through frequency of eating and the temperature of food and beverages consumed. The body's response to a cold environment is to maintain temperature by shivering, which will produce internal heat, and by constricting blood vessels so that heat cannot easily escape through the extremities; however, this comes with an increased calorie cost to the body and increased frequency of urination (figure 9.4).

Shivering causes an increase in RMR. As a result, there is an increased reliance on fat as the fuel source at rest; if the body continues shivering for a period of greater than 2 hours, an increase in carbohydrate will also be necessary to fuel the body. This is a result of muscular contraction, which is necessary to continue shivering and maintain the production of heat. For most athletes, this would occur only if warm insulating clothing was not worn during training in cold conditions; however, for mountaineers who spend long periods of time on expeditions in cold weather, this is a reality and must be accounted for by an increase in energy intake.

Dehydration in a cold environment is not uncommon. It occurs as a result of a decreased drive to drink, increased frequency of urination, increased water loss as a result of an increased frequency of breathing and the air being dry, and increased sweating from layers of clothing. The increase in urination is a result of **vasoconstriction** and thus an increased pressure throughout the body. This is dealt with by reducing the volume of blood through water losses in urine. As a result, athletes need to continually drink throughout the day. In the cold, this is best facilitated by keeping warm or hot beverages near the athlete's training site; when not at training, the athlete should aim to consume at least 4 ounces (120 ml) of fluid every 20 minutes throughout the day. This will help offset the decreased drive to drink in cold weather and the increased level of urination that may also be promoting an additional level of dehydration.

vasoconstriction – The narrowing of a blood vessel because of contraction of the muscular wall. This decreases blood flow through the vessel that is constricted.

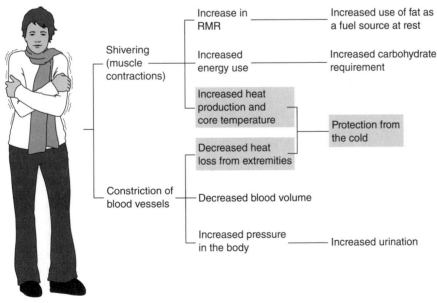

Cold exposure

Figure 9.4 Physical and metabolic reactions to cold.

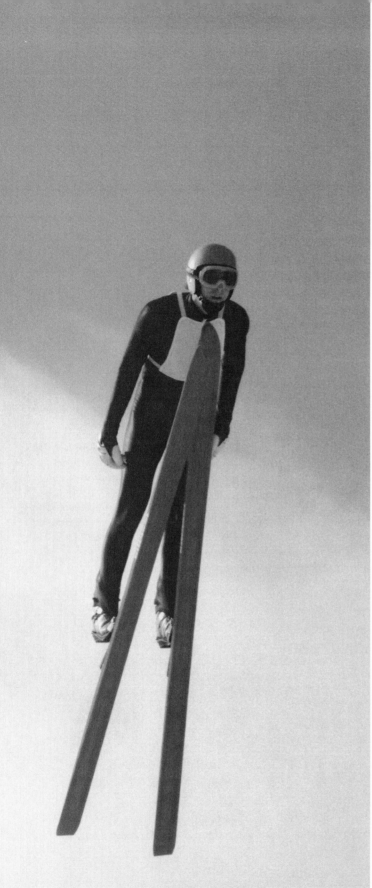

Athletes who train in cold environments must increase food and fluid intakes to account for increased RMR and frequency of urination.

During exercise in a cold environment, there is an increased metabolic cost. This can be attributed to decreased muscle efficiency and a decrease in blood volume; for some athletes, the weight of their clothing may also increase the amount of energy necessary to train. A muscle's efficiency is dependent on its temperature being within a range that allows for optimal muscle crossbridge formation. When a muscle is cooler than this range, it becomes less efficient at producing force. As a result, there is an increased reliance on carbohydrate because more muscle fibers need to be recruited to sustain work capacity. Lactate values are therefore usually higher during work in cold temperatures, indicating an increased reliance on anaerobic metabolism.

The other factor that causes an increased reliance on carbohydrate is the decrease in blood volume. When blood volume is decreased, the amount of blood that can be pumped per contraction of the heart is reduced. As a result, heart rate increases, and thus an athlete will be working at a greater relative percentage of maximal capacity. This again emphasizes the importance of maintaining hydration in a cold environment.

Training in the cold requires increased food and fluid intake. In this scenario, it is best to continue eating at least every 2 hours (if not more frequently) and increase food intake at each interval. Under these circumstances, no one macronutrient will assist more than any other; rather, it is simply maintaining energy stores that is important. Creating a timeline that promotes and allows for continual fluid ingestion is necessary to avoid dehydration.

Air Pollution

Air pollution is an environmental stress that can significantly affect the respiratory and cardiovascular systems of the body. **Pollutants** in the air can irritate the lungs and as a result reduce their capacity, increase breathing rate, and thus decrease oxygen supply to the body, resulting in a decreased performance capability. In addition, pollutants can decrease the ability to transport oxygen. When a pollutant enters the body, it has the potential to block the oxygen-binding sites on hemoglobin (the oxygen-carrying cell of the body) and thus diminish oxygen's ability to bind and be transported in the blood to exercising muscles. Once a pollutant enters the blood, it also has the potential to reach the brain. In turn, the brain may send messages to the body that minimize exercise capacity so that additional harm is not done to the body. In addition, pollutants can also trigger allergies and asthma, which will exacerbate the conditions of the respiratory system.

When a pollutant causes irritation of the lungs and nasal pathways, **inflammation** will occur within the body. This is magnified during exercise because the pollutant can reach deeper portions of the lungs. Exposure to pollution is often associated with the development of exercise-induced asthma (EIA). This results in constriction of the lungs so that air exchange cannot occur adequately, and therefore maximal exercise intensity cannot be reached. Inflammation will greatly tax the immune system and thus antioxidant status. Athletes attempt to minimize inflammation because it decreases the body's ability to recover and can cause damage to organs and tissues. The use of natural anti-inflammatories is potentially beneficial for athletes, especially when they are chronically pushing the upper limits of the body's capacity.

Two key strategies can help minimize EIA and assist the body in coping with high levels of inflammation. The first strategy is the use of fish oils. A 5.2-gram dose (3.2 grams of eicosapentaenoic acid and 2.0 grams of docosahexaenoic acid) has significant anti-inflammatory properties and helps prevent EIA and minimize the inflammation that can occur from pollutants. It can be taken in one dose or spread out across three time periods within the day, typically for a three-week period before exposure to air pollutants. The second strategy is to increase the intake of the antioxidant vitamins C and E. Doses of 500 to 1,500 mg of vitamin C and 100 mg of vitamin E have been shown to reduce the amount of stress the body experiences in polluted environments. Both of these strategies are even more beneficial for athletes with moderate to severe asthma.

pollutant – A contaminant in the environment that has the potential to cause discomfort to some portion of the physical body.

inflammation – A process in the body whereby white blood cells, antioxidants, and other chemicals protect tissues from free radicals and other damaging substances (e.g., viruses, bacteria).

Conclusion

The body's ability to adapt to stressful environments is highly dependent on sustaining energy, which can be used to maintain homeostasis. Acclimatization to an environment is a key component to ensure that athletes can perform without suffering the additional impact that an environment can cause. In the environments of heat, cold, and altitude, thirst and hunger should be avoided to ensure that health and performance are not compromised. Through creating a timing system that allows for a steady and constant flow of energy and fluid to the body's operating systems, athletes can significantly minimize the potential impacts of a stressful environment.

Case **Study**

Managing Dizziness and GI Distress

This case study describes an elite male triathlete in his late 30s. He focuses mostly on Olympic-distance (a 1.5 km swim, 40 km bike, and 10 km run) and half Ironman (a 1.2-mile swim, 56-mile bike, and 13.1-mile run) races.

BACKGROUND OF SPECIFIC ISSUES RELATIVE TO NUTRITION

In the past, he has experienced significant bouts of dizziness and GI distress, and he has a high sweat rate. He did not want to stop racing in warmer environments; he wanted to minimize and, if possible, completely eliminate the physical and nutritional issues he was having during racing.

NUTRITION GOAL

His main goals were to alleviate the feelings of dizziness he has when racing in warmer weather, significantly reduce or completely get rid of his GI distress, and improve his hydration status to counter his high sweat rate.

NUTRITION PLAN

Because this athlete had three nutrition challenges, each issue was approached independently. Often nutrition challenges are interrelated, but in this case the most important and detrimental to him, the dizziness spells, was selected as the first area to focus on. Getting dizzy during a race can be life threatening for a triathlete, especially if it happens on the bike as it was in this case. The first pieces of foundation nutrition reviewed were his overall daily eating plan and his balance of blood sugar. This would identify whether he was in poor control of his blood glucose and if his daily eating program had anything to do with these dizzy spells he was having during competitions. After he completed a food log of what, when, and why he ate throughout the day, it was clear that he was doing a very good job of eating a balance of carbohydrate, protein, and fat while staying adequately hydrated. Normal dietary habits were ruled out as a primary cause of his dizziness; however, it was noticed that he ate a very clean diet, meaning that he did not consume many processed or refined foods and therefore had a low daily intake of salt. A low-sodium diet will lower blood pressure in some athletes, and the lowered pressure can produce symptoms of dizziness at times, so monitoring sodium intake was a high priority.

The next issue to address was the challenge of GI distress. As any athlete can attest, GI distress of any kind is not enjoyable, and athletes will do whatever it takes to reduce the symptoms. With this athlete specifically, he was experiencing frequent bathroom breaks consisting of watery stools. Because it takes between 24 and 72 hours for a foodstuff to exit the body after entry, he was instructed to look at his daily eating regimen in the one to three days before competition. Common culprits that could increase the risk of GI distress include spicy foods; high-fiber foods; and any food or drink out of the ordinary because of travel, unfamiliar water sources, or new foods. He did very well with his prerace nutrition, and there were no red flags. Turning to his daily nutrition, he realized that his fat intake was fairly low. One low nutrient usually means another is too high, and in the case of endurance athletes, that nutrient is usually starchy carbohydrate that is higher in fiber. This could be a cause of GI distress. By increasing his daily fat intake slightly in the form of olive oil, nuts, and avocado, and thus creating a better balance of macronutrients, and by reducing his caloric intake while training and racing, he was able to completely get rid of the GI issues he was having.

His final goal was improving his hydration status and preventing himself from losing too much fluid, which would have a negative impact on his performance. He was aware of his sweat rate and prepared his fluid intake accordingly. He religiously stuck to his hydration plan during competition, and thus his quantity and timing of fluid intake were not an issue. However, the carbohydrate concentration and the electrolyte status of the sports drinks he was using were cause for concern. Sodium chloride (salt) specifically will help the body retain more fluids and prevent a high degree of dehydration. He has not typically fared well in hot and humid conditions, so he approached this from three different strategies: (1) heat acclimation, (2) sodium chloride use during competitions, and (3) sodium chloride loading before competitions.

From a heat acclimation standpoint, he tried to get accustomed to the heat and humidity whenever he could, 6 to 14 days before traveling to a warmer climate. This was not always possible depending on his schedule, so he did some cycling on an indoor trainer at home and tried to acclimatize to and train in the heat. The ideal scenario is for an athlete to travel to the competition site 6 to 14 days beforehand and begin the acclimation process there, but since that is not always an option for athletes, making do at home is a necessity. Many athletes will dress in more layers or put a space heater and humidifier in a training room in an effort to acclimatize. Whatever the process, athletes should pay particularly close attention to hydration and electrolyte status with the more challenging environmental extremes.

Regarding the athlete's salt intake, his daily quantity of salt consumption before and during a race was analyzed. As mentioned earlier, he ate a clean daily diet low in salt. Some athletes implement a pseudo salt-loading regimen, which includes using more salt on foods and when cooking in the week leading up to a race. This method may work for a only a small majority of athletes without GI distress symptoms, specifically bloating. To minimize the bloating response, he increased his salt intake immediately before his competitions. Through use of an electrolyte supplement, he consumed approximately 600 to 700 mg of sodium in the couple hours before a race. This low amount of an acute sodium load reduced his symptoms of fatigue and improved his hydration status without causing unnecessary bloating in the days leading up to the race. His normal salt intake during competitions varied depending on the conditions but normally ranged from 800 to 1,000 mg per hour. Because of his high sweat rate and sodium chloride being the main electrolyte lost in sweat, he implemented a higher salt intake during competitions, from 1,200 to 1,600 mg per hour. This was accomplished by choosing sports drinks rich in salt and, more important, by ingesting an electrolyte capsule that provided a higher amount of sodium specifically. His body's response to this was good. He felt better, and his bouts of dizziness lessened significantly. This led to him finishing his competitions without dropping out. In fact, he won one of them.

Competition Day

A large range of nutrients is needed during the competition cycle, and the preparation for and purpose of competition day are dependent on whether the event is of minimal, moderate, or significant importance. In addition, preparing for competition day is highly influenced by the type of athlete, the duration of the taper, how significantly training volume and intensity are reduced to prepare for the event, and how the body adapts to overcome any fatigue from training. Most important is that the athlete rest as much as possible and ensure the body is as full of energy sources as it can be.

Preparing for competition day starts with the first day of an athlete's taper. For major competitions, most athletes use a four-day to four-week taper that progressively reduces training volume but maintains intensity. Depending on the sport, some athletes will need to consciously watch their food intake to ensure weight gain does not occur, while others may just need to be aware that food intake should be slightly reduced in relation to volume and intensity of training for each day's effort. The goal should be to focus on supporting training with carbohydrate and providing sufficient protein to ensure the body is repairing tissues. Hydration is also a key component to feeling mentally and physically sound. If you are an athlete, ensuring that you enjoy the food you eat is important to support a happy and healthy mind-set going into competition.

The goal for any minor and moderate competitions is to come into the event as rested as possible and also simulate what will occur at a major competition. Athletes should take these opportunities to ensure that the game plan for the day of major competition and days leading into competition is sound. This should include evaluating what foods digest well, how far in advance of the day's competition the food needs to be consumed, the frequency of eating throughout the competition day, how much fiber should be in the diet, and how much fluid will be needed to ensure good hydration.

The remainder of this chapter is devoted to case study examples of how athletes can best prepare for the day of competition. The case studies are divided into the sport classifications described previously: acrobatic and combative, strength and power, endurance, and team and technical sports.

Combative Sports (Weight Classified)

Combative sports include taekwondo, wrestling, judo, boxing, and mixed martial arts, among others. These sports are classified by weight in an attempt to equalize the competitors' size. Athletes are required to achieve the weight for their sport at the time of weigh-in. Depending on the sport and level of competitor, this may be anywhere from 30 minutes to 18 hours or more before the matches begin. Sports such as boxing at the Olympic and world championship levels require repeated days in which the athlete must make weight before each fight. The example here shows how to design a competition-day plan for a wrestler at the national level. This same system can be applied to other weight-classified sports because they share commonalities in energy needs. The main differences will be the length of time between weigh-ins and competition and the logistics of the competition (e.g., spread over multiple days or a single day).

Sport: Wrestling, Weight Classified

Competition details: There are three different primary forms of wrestling: Greco, freestyle, and folk. At the national and international levels, Greco and freestyle are the forms of competition, and at the high school and collegiate levels, athletes compete in folk. Each round of a wrestling match includes three 2-minute bouts with approximately 30 seconds of recovery between bouts. Most wrestlers at the national and international levels train and live at a higher weight than they fight at. As long as weigh-in occurs in the day before competition, athletes at this level will always use some form of weight cutting. This is because there is a direct correlation between strength and the cross section of muscle size. An increase in muscle size (and therefore mass) results in an increase in strength.

Athletes should compete in a weight class that allows for optimal body composition while also taking into consideration the height and weight of their competitors. Research examining cognitive function, muscle function in various states of hydration, and glycogen depletion and restoration suggests that a weight cut of 5 to 8 percent of body weight is feasible when in a fully hydrated state. An athlete should develop a protocol that will effectively reduce body weight without compromising performance. A weight-cutting protocol should last no more than five days and ideally no more than three. At the national and international levels, athletes weigh in on the afternoon before competition and typically have about 18 hours to recover. For high school and collegiate athletes, weigh-in occurs the day of competition, with one to two hours between weigh-in and start of the match. Weight cut recommendations for these two scenarios are shown in figure 10.1. Developing a timeline of fluid, electrolyte, and carbohydrate intake to facilitate recovery from strategies used to make weight is a key aspect of competing successfully in wrestling.

Regardless of wrestling style, competition begins late morning, and for the successful competitor, rounds continue every 30 minutes to 2 hours throughout the day. The typical competition day is approximately 8 hours long. This requires athletes to have a nutrition plan that optimizes the timing of food and fluid intake so that energy is available for each match and does not result in the stomach being too full for competition.

Energy systems used: Wrestling relies on both the ATP–CP and anaerobic glycolysis pathways to supply the energy needed for repeated maximal bouts of power and speed. Recovery is facilitated through all the energy systems.

Nutrition goals leading up to competition: The main goal heading into competition for any weight-classified athlete is to safely make weight without compromising health and performance. When athletes must weigh in on the day of competition, it is recommended that they compete at the weight class that allows for the most natural body weight in a fully hydrated state. This is best achieved by losing excess body weight in the off-season and early preseason, losing no more than 5 percent of body weight through dehydration in the 24 hours leading up to competition, and losing up to 3 percent through food restriction in the 48 hours before competition for a total of 8 percent of body weight throughout the three days leading into competition.

- Reduction of body weight by up to 5 percent can be accomplished through dehydration. This is highly dependent on an athlete's sweat rate and ability to tolerate the chosen method of dehydration. It is also beneficial to acclimate to heat (such as that experienced in a sauna) before using it for competition dehydration. This can be achieved over a 14-day period before competition or by intermittent use of the sauna throughout the year on light training days.

- Research shows that over a three-day period, body weight can be reduced by up to 3 percent through food restriction and exercise that depletes glycogen stores. Exercise should not be overly intense so that muscle fatigue is an issue.

- Reducing fiber in the diet can help minimize weight; however, the diet should still be made up of mainly carbohydrate. Foods should be low in residue, and up to 50 percent of caloric intake can come from liquid meals.

Timeline

Nutrition Timeline for a Wrestler's Weight-Cutting Protocol

- **3 days before competition:** Athlete begins consuming low-residue foods.
- **2 days before competition:** Athlete begins caloric restriction if necessary. This should be no more than 50 percent of usual caloric intake. Ensure good hydration with electrolytes.
- **1 day before competition:** Same as 2 days before.
- **12 hours before competition:** Dehydration of 3 percent body mass.
- **2 hours before competition:** Athlete should be at weight and have recovery foods that are ready to go. Weigh-ins should occur shortly.
- **1 hour before competition:** Weigh-ins should have occurred, and the athlete should be consuming a carbohydrate–electrolyte beverage for rehydration and fueling. This may also include intake of salty foods such as pretzels and saltines. The goal is to regain approximately 2 percent of body mass before competition.
- **During competition:** The athlete should utilize a nibbling and sipping protocol of previously identified sports drinks and low-glycemic foods that will help maintain hydration and blood glucose levels.

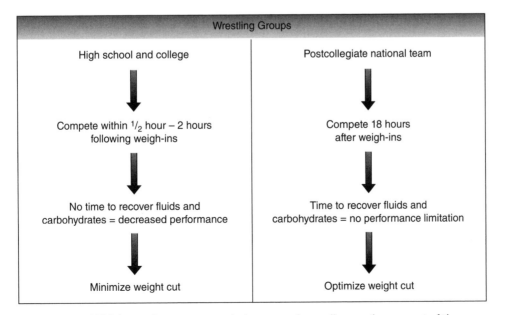

Figure 10.1 Weight-cutting recommendations vary depending on the amount of time between weigh-in and competition. For wrestlers at the high school and college levels, this typically means weight cut should be minimal.

Heat Acclimation for Weight Cutting

A collegiate wrestler was 10 weeks out from his first competition of the year. He had certified for the weight class of 125 pounds (57 kg) earlier that year but had done so by cutting weight. At this point he was 138 pounds (63 kg) and knew he not only needed to lose weight but also needed to make weight by cutting no more than 5 percent of his body mass. The nutritionist advised that he begin to lose .5 to 1 pound (.2 to .5 kg) per week by consuming five or six meals per day that contained 50 percent of the calories as fruits and vegetables, 30 percent as protein, and the remainder as whole grains. The athlete also worked on becoming well hydrated by drinking continually throughout the day. Weight loss stopped at least two weeks before the competition so his body had a chance to regenerate. Over the eight-week period, the athlete was able to lose six pounds (2.7 kg) without compromising his training. He then stabilized his body weight for the next two weeks so that the weight cut was feasible and easy to achieve.

The athlete would make weight by following this formula:

low-residue foods + slight food restriction + float weight + dehydration.

He would need to cut a total of 7 pounds (3.2 kg). By eating low-residue foods, the athlete lost 1 pound (.5 kg); cutting food back by 25 percent resulted in another pound, and he had a 1-pound float even when dehydrated. In the evening before weighing in, he would sweat out the 4 remaining pounds (1.8 kg).

To make sure his body was prepared for the dehydration, the athlete used a heat-acclimation protocol of cycling while wearing long sleeves and sweats for 30 to 60 minutes a day for two weeks prior to the week before competition. He did this after practice so as not to disturb his readiness for training. His recovery after the cycling sessions included cooling his body and rehydrating with a carbohydrate–electrolyte beverage for 30 minutes. This would be similar to the time he would have to recover before competing. He then continued to sip on the beverage all evening to mimic how he could stay hydrated during competition. In the last week before his competition, the athlete did not do the cycling to give his body a break.

- Ideally, the athlete's diet includes five or six meals per day; two or three should be in liquid form and three would be composed of low-residue foods.
- The athlete should reduce meal size over the next five days, progressively moving to lesser amounts (three-quarters, two-thirds, one-half).
- On the day before weigh-in, the athlete may want to dehydrate by 2 percent of body weight in the afternoon training session by maximizing fluid lost as sweat. On the day of weigh-in, dehydration up to an additional 3 percent can be accomplished. After weigh-in, athletes should begin an aggressive nutrition recovery plan.
- The recovery plan should focus on recovering fluid, electrolytes, and carbohydrate stores. A significant key to refeeding is food variety. Fluid replacement must be 1.5 times the amount lost in sweat, and the athlete should consume at least the following in the immediate 2.5 hours after weigh-in. This can best be achieved by consuming at least 20 percent of the suggested intake below every 30 minutes:
  - 9.5 calories per pound (21 cal/kg)
  - 15 mg sodium per pound (33 mg/kg)
  - 13 ml of fluid per pound (29 ml/kg) (at least)

- Water can be consumed freely as desired to further facilitate fluid replacement. At least half the fluids consumed should have electrolytes, and water should be consumed around food.

- The athlete should let the food settle after the initial recovery feeding and then focus on dinner. Dinner should be rich in starchy carbohydrate, with adequate protein and minimal fiber. The meal should not be so large that the athlete eats past full. He should still focus on consuming additional noncarbonated fluids and water.

Competition Day

Competition-day nutrition is very individual and depends on what sits best with the athlete when needing to compete. The following are general recommendations to assist in determining food type and timing for competition:

- Breakfast should be moderate to high in carbohydrate, moderate to low in protein, and low in fat and fiber. The amount eaten depends on how full the stomach feels and should not leave the athlete feeling heavy.

- For the remainder of the day, the athlete can snack on a variety of low-residue foods every 30 to 60 minutes, even if it is a very small amount.

- Athletes should identify the carbohydrate–electrolyte beverage that tastes best to them and practice using it before, during, and after training. The goal is to figure out how much can be consumed in the hour before, every 15 minutes during, and in the hour after training. This should allow the athlete to develop a timeline that can be applied to competition. For most athletes, this will allow for 16 to 20 ounces (480 to 600 ml) of fluid in the hour before competition begins; gulps or sips between rounds of competition; and depending on the time between rounds, 4 to 24 ounces (120 to 720 ml) in the 30 minutes to 2 hours after competing.

- After competition is completed for the day, it is important that the athlete have a carbohydrate and protein snack within 30 minutes of finishing and a meal within 2 hours. This meal should focus on moderate carbohydrate and protein intake and be low in fat and fiber. The athlete should also focus on continuing to hydrate and replace fluids that have been lost as sweat.

Timeline

Postcompetition Recovery Timeline for a Wrestler

- **Less than 45 minutes after competition:** Carbohydrate and protein beverage containing at least .5 grams of carbohydrate per kilogram of body weight and at least 6 grams of protein

- **Less than 2 hours after competition:** Low- to moderate-glycemic meal to assist in refueling

- **More than 2 hours after competition:** Nibbling based on hunger; milk or a similar beverage before sleeping

Strength and Power Sports

Strength and power sports include swimming, powerlifting, track and field, skiing, and kayaking. These sports are dominated by the anaerobic energy systems and are evaluated based on some measure of physical capacity. This measure may be the amount of time it takes to cover a set distance or the amount of power that can be generated to move an object (e.g., shotput) or large amount of weight (e.g., powerlifting). These sports frequently require successful athletes to go through multiple rounds of competition. In some instances, such as track and field, skiing, and swimming, athletes may also choose to compete in more than one event and as a result will compete on consecutive days.

Sport: Track and Field, Sprints and Hurdles

Competition details: There are six sprint and hurdle events: 100 meters, 100/110-meter hurdles, 200 meters, 400 meters, 400-meter hurdles, and 800 meters. Athletes frequently compete in meets where there is just one round of the event, but they must also be prepared to compete in single- and multiple-day competitions. Most athletes will peak for national and world championship meets, where rounds carried out over multiple days qualify athletes for the final competition.

An athlete's start time can be quite varied. It will usually be in the afternoon but can be as late as 9:00 p.m. At high school, collegiate, national, and world championship events, up to two rounds for some events can occur within the day. Rounds are traditionally at least 2 hours apart as athletes qualify for the next day or finals. Some athletes may choose to compete in more than one event, and whether this is feasible often depends on how the track meet is designed. Events are hopefully separated by days so an athlete does not need to compete in two events within the same day. At the most, an athlete may compete in the final of one event and the initial rounds of the second event on the same day. Depending on the setup of the competition, an athlete needs to have a flexible program so nutrient timing can easily be manipulated to accommodate any schedule.

Energy systems used: The energy system used is dependent on the sprint distance. The 100 meters and 100/110-meter hurdles rely on the ATP–CP energy system for power and speed. The 200 meters, 400 meters, 800 meters, and 400-meter hurdles use both the ATP–CP and anaerobic glycolysis energy systems. Recovery is facilitated by all the energy systems.

Nutrition goals leading up to competition: The primary goals during the competitive season for sprint and hurdle athletes are maintaining a stable body weight and minimizing the sensations of fatigue and heaviness that can come from multiple competitions and traveling as well as ensuring the foods they eat have adequate energy for competing and will not induce GI distress. This involves planning well in advance of travel as well as exploring what will be available at the destination. Food needs to be wholesome and remain as consistent as possible. All too frequently, athletes will stop at fast-food restaurants or just eat what is available at the meet. This usually is not appropriate for sustaining a high level of competitive readiness; preparations should be made before leaving on a trip. If you are an athlete, the following suggestions will help you prepare to compete frequently and with a significant travel schedule:

- Wear compression stockings to help minimize edema that can potentially occur while traveling.
- Pack appropriate snack foods, and carry them throughout the trip.

- Research the area being traveled to, and determine food availability. Identify key foods to take with you, restaurants and grocery stores near the hotel and the training and competition facilities, and whether you can prepare food in the hotel room (microwave, electrical outlets, access to purified water).

- Create a timeline for consuming food and fluids throughout the day—and stick to it. This will help ensure you are not overeating or forgetting to eat as you travel and that you travel, train, and compete in a hydrated state.

Competition Day

The type and amount of food an athlete can consume on the day of competition is very individualized. Some athletes can remain calm going into competition, while others can be quite nervous. In events such as the sprints and hurdles, some athletes may even desire an increase in alertness and energy. Since competition usually starts later in the day, most athletes should begin by consuming a normal breakfast and then continuing to snack throughout the day on foods that they know will function well for them. The following are some recommendations to assist in planning for competition:

- Create a timeline for consuming food that can be tried in training or at a smaller competition. The timeline should come from the schedule used at most of the athlete's competitions and should provide some level of food intake at least every 3 hours. Fluids should be consumed consistently throughout the day.

- In the case of competing in multiple rounds or over multiple days, it is important that athletes consume a postrace snack that provides carbohydrate and protein to sustain energy and preserve muscle glycogen stores while also minimizing fat and fiber intake. Athletes should optimally consume a meal within 2 hours of completing the last race of the day. The sooner an athlete can begin to recover, the better prepared they can be to compete the next day or at the next meet.

- Identify foods that are easily consumed regardless of the athlete's emotional and psychological state. These foods should be ones that are familiar to the athlete and can be consumed without leaving a feeling of fullness in the stomach. Frequently foods that are low in residue are most easily digested. The goal is to maintain stable blood glucose levels, supply a constant line of energy, and avoid any GI distress that may result from nervousness. The following common snack foods can be easily transported and consumed:

  o Fruit twists or fruit leather

  o Half a sandwich on white bread

  o Low-fat muffins

  o Cereal or sports bars

- Hydration status and electrolyte balance should be maintained by carrying two bottles of fluid, one with water and the other with sports drink or another fluid that contains the electrolytes sodium and potassium.

Time Line

Competition-Day Nutrition Timeline for a Sprinter or Hurdler

- **More than 2 hours before competition:** Low-glycemic breakfast such as oatmeal with peanut butter and skim milk plus banana

- **Less than 2 hours before competition:** Low-glycemic carbohydrate–electrolyte beverage

- **Less than 1 hour before competition:** Sipping on fluids that contain some form of carbohydrates and electrolytes

- **During competition:** Nibbling on foods and sipping on fluids based on hunger; foods should be low glycemic such as half a turkey sandwich, Greek yogurt with fruit, 4 to 8 oz (120 to 240 ml) smoothie with protein

- **Less than 45 minutes after competition:** Carbohydrate and protein snack containing at least .5 grams of carbohydrate per kilogram of body weight and at least 6 grams of protein

- **Less than 2 hours after competition:** Low-glycemic meal eaten until full (e.g., a chicken salad, half a sandwich with soup, a stir-fry)

- **More than 2 hours after competition:** Continued nibbling and sipping based on hunger; again foods should be low glycemic such as banana with almond butter, apple with low-fat cheese, cup of melon with feta cheese, cottage cheese and fruit, Greek yogurt with seeds

Endurance Sports

Endurance sports cover a variety of events consisting of short-duration (under 2 hours) to multiday competitions and include sports such as running, triathlon, cycling, rowing, canoeing and kayaking, swimming, biathlon, and cross-country skiing. Each endurance sport has its own individual nutrient timing challenges based on the intensity and duration of the competition. A short- and long-course triathlon provides a good overall example of how to implement a nutrient timing system within an endurance sport. Although the sport is triathlon, the system can be applied to many other endurance-classified sports because they share commonalities in energy needs. The main differences will be the length and the logistics of the competition.

Sport: Triathlon, Short and Long Distances

Competition details: There are four main distances in the sport of triathlon. Sprint-distance triathlon races typically involve a quarter- to half-mile swim, 12- to 18-mile bike ride, and 3.1-mile run. The Olympic-distance triathlon includes a 1.5-kilometer swim followed by a 40-kilometer bike ride (in a drafting or nondrafting format) followed by a 10-kilometer run. Half Ironman triathlons involve a 1.2-mile swim, a 56-mile bike ride, and a 13.1-mile run. Ironman triathlons involve a 2.4-mile swim, 112-mile bike ride, and 26.2-mile run (1 mile = 1.6 kilometers). Competition times greatly depend on the level of athlete, with professionals and elite age-groupers recording faster times and recreational and beginning athletes registering slower times. Sprint-distance events last approximately 55 minutes to 1 hour and 30 minutes, Olympic distances from 1 hour and 45 minutes to 3 hours, half Ironman distances from just under 4 hours to 7 hours, and Ironman distances from just under 8 hours to 17 hours. For recreational triathletes, racing usually begins early in the morning, between 6:00 and 8:00 a.m. Professional triathletes

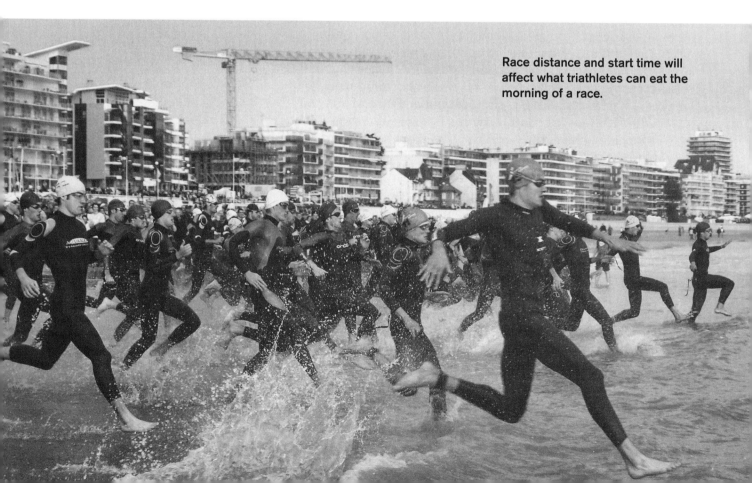

Race distance and start time will affect what triathletes can eat the morning of a race.

competing in Olympic draft-legal races often start racing later, between 11:00 a.m. and 3:00 p.m. Each event poses different nutrition challenges in terms of nutrient timing.

Energy systems used: The aerobic energy system predominates, but it is important to note that all energy systems are relied on during some events, especially during the start.

Nutrition goals leading up to competition: The main goals for most triathletes include reducing GI distress, maintaining adequate hydration and electrolyte levels, and not gaining weight due to a decrease in energy expenditure during their taper.

The taper itself presents a significant challenge for triathletes. Because the range of the taper is large—4 to 28 days depending on the coach and distance—athletes do not often know how to navigate the time leading up to competition, and thus water retention and feelings of bloating and heaviness are common. Eating will depend somewhat on the length of the taper, but triathletes can use the following nutrition goals:

- Increasing daily salt intake is usually a common practice during the taper, but athletes should try this during quality training sessions well before the race because it sometimes leads to slight bloating and water weight gain.

- A two- or three-day fiber taper can be extremely beneficial for some triathletes who are more susceptible to GI distress or have a sensitive gut. It is recommended to decrease fiber intake by 25 percent each day two or three days out from the race by focusing on more white starch products and juices.

- Maintaining hydration status is important, and overdrinking water is a common practice. If water is used as the primary fluid throughout the day, salty foods should be eaten at the same time in an effort to prevent hyponatremia. It is also recommended that triathletes drink when thirsty and not try to hyperhydrate with water leading up to the race.

- Maintaining energy levels is crucial during the taper so that the craving response is reduced. In an effort to stabilize blood glucose levels, triathletes should combine a source of lean protein, healthy fat, a fruit or vegetable, and a starch during all feedings. Triathletes should avoid eating only a starch by itself because it will raise blood glucose levels quickly and could lead to overeating during the taper.

- Stabilizing body weight is a primary goal of all triathletes leading up to a race, and as mentioned previously, this is typically difficult to control because of decreases in training volume. Athletes should not overeat and try to overcompensate their caloric intake in an effort to load before competition. Most athletes who follow a balanced eating program consisting of moderate carbohydrate, moderate protein, and low to moderate fat should continue this type of eating during their taper. Frequency of eating may be a variable that triathletes can consider changing, meaning they may not need to eat as many times throughout the day. Eating to train during a taper becomes a good mantra to follow, and since training is reduced, so should food intake.

Timeline

Competition-Day Nutrition Timeline for a Triathlete

- **More than 2 hours before competition:** Small breakfast with moderate carbohydrate, moderate to low protein, and low fat, such as a bagel and thin layer of peanut butter, cereal or oatmeal with skim milk, low-fat yogurt and juice, or an energy bar and sports drink

- **1 to 2 hours before competition:** Light snack such as a carbohydrate–electrolyte beverage; energy bars, gels, or chews; white bread with jelly; or fruit smoothie

- **Less than 1 hour before competition:** Sports drink with added electrolytes

- **During competition:** 3 to 8 oz (90 to 240 ml) of a sports drink every 15 to 30 minutes or water, electrolytes, and energy gel

- **Less than 45 minutes after competition:** Snack with higher carbohydrate, moderate protein, and minimal fat and fiber, such as a carbohydrate and protein recovery shake, skim milk fruit smoothie, or yogurt and fruit

- **More than 2 hours after competition:** A well-balanced meal consisting of carbohydrate, protein, and fat (specifically omega-3 or monounsaturated) 2 hours after the first postrace feeding; reintroduce fiber slowly if a fiber taper was used before the race

Competition Day

Race-day nutrition is highly individual for all triathletes, and the race distance and start time will dictate much of what a triathlete can consume the morning of a race. The following general recommendations pertain to early-morning races:

- A smaller breakfast made up of moderate carbohydrate, moderate to low protein, and low fat is recommended. A liquid snack or meal such as a smoothie may be beneficial for those who have very sensitive stomachs.

- Athletes should hydrate but should pay attention to not overhydrating with water alone as this can increase the risk of hyponatremia. Consuming water with salty foods or a sports drink with sodium is recommended.

- For athletes competing later in the day, a normal breakfast that has worked for the athlete during higher-intensity training can be eaten followed by an easily digestible snack 1 to 2 hours before the race. Liquid sources are typically preferred.

- After the race, it is common for athletes to forget about their nutrition. The postrace nutrition plan is crucial for allowing an athlete to replenish glycogen and fluid stores. The basic guidelines on what to eat in the first 15 to 60 minutes after a race include higher carbohydrate, moderate protein, and minimal fat and fiber. Athletes should plan ahead of time to ensure that foods or beverages are available after their race. After the initial feeding, athletes should try to eat well-balanced meals consisting of carbohydrate, protein, and fat (specifically omega-3 or monounsaturated) 2 hours after the first postrace feeding.

- If a fiber taper was implemented before a race, it is important to reintroduce fiber slowly into the normal daily nutrition plan by reversing the recommendations stated previously. That is, increase fiber gradually by 25 percent each day after the race to allow the body to get used to the normal amounts without causing GI distress.

Team Sports

Team sports such as soccer, football, basketball, and volleyball have specific nutrient timing challenges, most notably the inability to consume food and fluids at frequent intervals because of continuous play. These challenges are prominent during competition, and athletes in these sports must find appropriate fueling strategies to offset the logistics of the sport's rules.

Sport: Soccer

Competition details: Soccer is known as football in most countries outside the United States and Canada. Soccer games, often called matches, are played in two separate 45-minute halves with a 15-minute halftime. Players rarely get breaks during a match unless there is an injury; thus, the opportunities to refuel and rehydrate are minimal. This poses a significant challenge for athletes and stresses the importance of pregame nutrition and hydration. During the competitive season, athletes can play one to three games per week and often participate in multiple-game tournaments, sometimes playing matches within 1 to 2 hours of each other, adding more complexity to the nutrient timing plan.

Energy systems used: Soccer is unique in that there are times of sprinting, jogging, and no movement at all. For high-intensity sprints, both the anaerobic glycolysis and the ATP–CP energy systems contribute, but the ATP–CP system will be more important. Most soccer players train all three energy systems, paying particular attention to the ATP–CP and aerobic systems.

Nutrition goals leading up to competition: The main nutrition goals for most soccer players include having adequate stores of glycogen to fuel both the aerobic and higher-intensity times during a game. Hydration and electrolyte stores also become important because a single match can significantly deplete glycogen and fluids. Once fatigue starts to set in, speed, accuracy of ball placement, ball-handling skills, and concentration begin to decline, which will have a negative impact on performance. Muscle cramping and the risk of dehydration increase, especially in warmer and more humid environments. The following nutrition goals should be met before soccer matches:

- Athletes should eat sufficient carbohydrate in the daily nutrition plan leading up to the match and include good sources from fruits, vegetables, and whole grains. Eating these types of foods throughout the days of the competitive season will ensure adequate glycogen stores.

- Maintaining hydration status is crucial. Athletes must stay hydrated before the match and continually assess hydration status using one of the methods presented in chapter 5. The easiest way to stay hydrated is by carrying a fluid bottle around throughout the day and continually taking drinks out of it. As the match gets closer, switching to a sports drink can help improve hydration status and supply much-needed electrolytes.

Timeline

Competition-Day Nutrition Timeline for a Soccer Player

- **More than 2 hours before competition:** A breakfast with moderate to moderately high carbohydrate, moderate to low protein, and low fat, such as cereal, oatmeal, toast with peanut butter, milk-based fruit smoothie with one or two pinches of salt, or yogurt and granola; hydration either with water and salty foods or a sports drink

- **1 to 2 hours before competition:** Snack-size portion; good options include sports drink with carbohydrate and electrolytes; energy bars (higher in carbohydrate, moderate to low in protein, low in fat, and low in fiber); peanut butter and jelly or honey sandwich; fruit smoothie made with milk and fruit; or for more sensitive stomachs, fruit juice, protein powder, and a pinch of salt

- **Less than 1 hour before competition:** Water or sports drink

- **During competition:** Up to 10 oz (300 ml) of sports drink during halftime

- **Less than 60 minutes after competition:** Foods and beverages that are high in carbohydrate, moderate in protein, and very low in fat and fiber, such as a carbohydrate and protein recovery shake, lean-meat sandwich, yogurt and fruit, and energy or cereal bars

- **If another match is to be played in 1 to 3 hours:** Sports drink or smoothie and high-glycemic carbohydrate sources

- **More than 2 hours after competition:** Well-balanced meals consisting of carbohydrate, protein, and fat (specifically omega-3 or monounsaturated) every 2 to 3 hours after the first postmatch feeding

- If the match or tournament will be played in a hot and humid environment, athletes should add extra electrolytes, specifically sodium, to their normal eating program one or two days before the match. Easy ways of doing this are by choosing foods such as pretzels, crackers, pickles, olives, and lean deli meats for sandwiches and by adding salt to boiling water if pasta or rice is being cooked.

Competition Day

Soccer matches can begin in the morning or afternoon and sometimes the evening. This makes it challenging for some athletes to time their nutrition appropriately. The following are suggestions for matches played in the morning:

- A breakfast containing moderate to moderately high carbohydrate, moderate to low protein, and low fat should be eaten 2 to 4 hours before the match. As match time gets closer, the size of the meal should be reduced to allow for adequate digestion. Athletes are encouraged to maintain their normal prematch meal or snack choice as long as it adheres to these nutrient recommendations. Trying new foods and beverages the day of a match is not advised.

- Athletes should hydrate either with water and salty foods or a sports drink. Drinking plain water without salt will dilute the blood sodium and increase the risk of hyponatremia before the match.

- For matches later in the day, a normal breakfast can be eaten, but the remaining feedings should be smaller snack portions. This will help the food digest quicker and minimize the risk of GI distress.

- After the match, it is crucial to replenish glycogen and fluid stores since the athlete may either return to practice the following day or will be playing in another match later that day or the next during a tournament. The basic guidelines on what to eat in the first 15 to 60 minutes after a match focus on foods and beverages that are higher in carbohydrate, moderate in protein, and very low in fat and fiber. After the first postmatch feeding, athletes should try to eat well-balanced meals consisting of carbohydrate, protein, and fat (specifically omega-3 or monounsaturated) every 2 to 3 hours.

- If the athlete is playing in a tournament, rehydrating with a sports drink or smoothie and eating high-glycemic carbohydrate sources are the best bets to be ready for the next match if it is played 1 to 3 hours after the first.

Long-Duration Sports Requiring Concentration

Sports such as sailing often require a long duration of both physical activity and mental concentration associated with tactics. There are considerable nutrition challenges for athletes who sail, including finding easily digestible foods, watertight foods and beverages, ensuring the ease of opening and closing food products, and storage. All of these in addition to the duration of races will factor into a well-designed nutrition plan.

Sport: Sailing

Competition details: There are many disciplines in the sport of sailing, ranging from one-person to three-person boats. Competition days can range from 2 or 3 longer races (45 to 70 minutes) to 3 to 10 shorter races (10 to 25 minutes). Different energy systems will be used and different amounts of energy expended. Regardless of the quantity of races or duration of competition, sailors have extended periods of time on the water and require constant physical and mental energy. Maneuvering boats and playing a mental chess game against opponents requires a great deal of concentration. Additionally, sailors must closely monitor wind and water conditions and factor these variables into the overall tactical plan. Depending on the length of the competition, energy expenditure can be somewhat steady or more oscillating, with high amounts of energy used for short bursts of activity. Some classes require intense physical exertion and mental concentration. Sailing takes place year-round and does not often use a traditional taper as do other sports. Thus, sailors must be consistent with their nutrition plan in supporting their training cycles and competition plans throughout the year.

Energy systems used: Sailing can use a blend of all energy systems depending on the duration and specific competition class.

Nutrition goals leading up to competition: Weight goals vary among the different classes of boats; some athletes require weight gain to improve performance, while others seek weight loss. One of the most important nutrition goals leading up to competition day is to achieve the desired body weight for optimal performance.

For sailors seeking to gain weight for performance reasons, the daily nutrition plan must include more nutrient-dense foods throughout the day, timed with their training. Increasing the overall caloric load of the day is important, and easy ways to do this include the following:

- Adding extra-virgin olive oil to meals and snacks such as smoothies, oatmeal, yogurt, salads, sauces, pasta, and rice
- Including a high-calorie super smoothie (e.g., add peanut butter to milk and banana with whey protein isolate powder, or frozen yogurt to a milk-based smoothie)
- Eating protein with carbohydrate in the 30 to 60 minutes before an interval or strength training session and again in the 30 to 60 minutes after training to maintain positive protein stores and provide extra fuel for the body to perform the workout
- Adding a few extra bites to each meal or snack
- Adding an after-dinner snack consisting of protein and carbohydrate (Greek yogurt with berries, a bowl of cereal with fruit, or a whole-grain bagel with peanut butter are good options)

Although eating foods high in fiber supports overall health, athletes who are trying to gain weight may not be able to eat enough calories throughout the day because of the high satiety feeling. Thus, keeping fiber at moderate levels during times of weight gain is one key to success while including other foods higher in calories.

For athletes seeking weight loss, improving satiety through a balance of lean protein, healthy fat, fruits and vegetables, and whole grains becomes the goal. Eating in this manner will introduce a lower daily caloric load. Eating to stabilize blood sugar and insulin through the proper combinations of foods is the most important factor. Additionally, not using calorie-containing sports nutrition products that do not support energy expenditure is a key factor in losing weight during training.

Competition Day

The competition day normally begins early, around 8:00 or 9:00 in the morning for weather briefings and meetings with coaches. Athletes leave the dock shortly thereafter and head out on the water to wait for competition to begin. The start of competition can be 1 to 2 hours after the athletes leave the dock. Once competition begins, athletes are faced with refueling and rehydrating challenges based on the degree of energy expenditure from their races and the ability to store foods and beverages on their boats; foods must be palatable and nonperishable and must elicit a

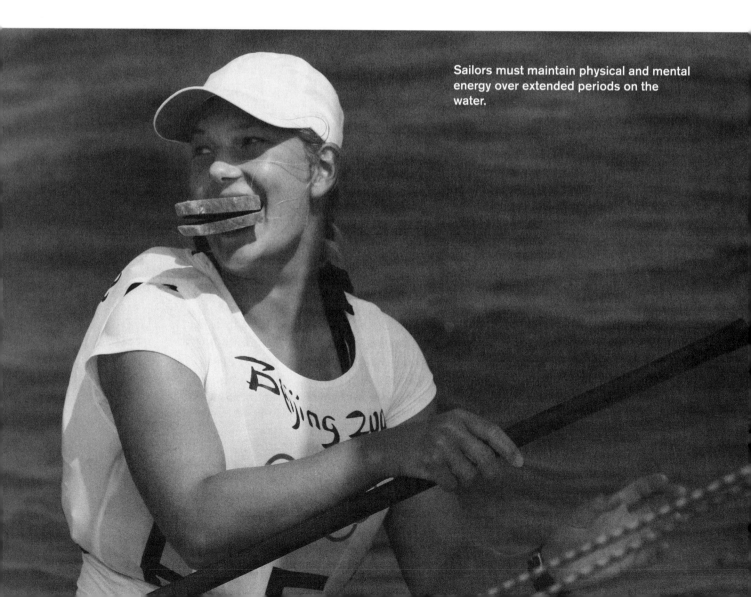

Sailors must maintain physical and mental energy over extended periods on the water.

steady blood sugar response. The latter is of extreme importance because if energy level ebbs and flows during a race, performance will decline significantly. Thus, finding proper combinations of foods and beverages while on the water is of utmost importance.

- Beginning the day with a hearty nutrient-balanced meal is a top goal so that athletes enter their competition day with stable blood sugar levels.

- Sailing competitions can last from 4 to 8 hours, during which time athletes can become malnourished and dehydrated quite quickly. Because race times can depend on weather, it is somewhat difficult to prescribe an exact nutrient timing system. However, carbohydrate, fluid, and electrolyte intake is primary, with the addition of protein as a blood sugar stabilizer for longer events as a secondary goal while on the water. It is usually recommended, based on competition timing, that sailors try to consume smaller amounts of food and adequate fluids and electrolytes between races.

- After competition, sailors will return to the dock and derig their boats before debriefing with their coaches. The amount of time from the cessation of competition to the next meal (dinner) can be upwards of 3 to 4 hours; thus planning and preparing a snack for the postcompetition time frame is extremely important to begin the nutrition recovery process. Because sailors will be breaking down their boats for up to an hour after they finish competing, it is best that they eat some type of light snack to begin the rehydration and nourishment process. Ready-to-drink fruit smoothies, natural energy bars, and yogurt with fruit along with adequate fluid intake can all provide the nutrients to jump-start the nutrition recovery process until athletes can have a full meal a couple of hours later.

- Once dinner is eaten, it is recommended that athletes consume a balance of carbohydrate and protein with lower amounts of healthy fat; alcohol intake should be avoided or limited, especially if another competition will be held the next day.

Timeline

Competition-Day Nutrition Timeline for a Sailor

- **More than 2 hours before competition:** A hearty nutrient-balanced meal that will sustain blood sugar levels throughout the morning, including a balance of carbohydrate, protein, and healthy fat along with adequate fluids

- **Less than 2 hours before competition:** Light snack consisting of carbohydrate, protein, and healthy fat (e.g., a fruit smoothie with whey protein isolate powder or milk, yogurt with berries, or an energy bar with water)

- **Less than 1 hour before competition:** Sports drink to provide fluid and electrolytes

- **During competition:** Carbohydrate, fluid, and electrolytes with the addition of protein as a blood sugar stabilizer; some foods that work for nutrition on the water include peanut butter and jelly or honey sandwiches; energy bars that have a more balanced nutrient profile of carbohydrate, protein, and fat; and trail mix

- **Less than 2 hours after competition:** Fruit smoothies, natural energy bars, and yogurt with fruit along with adequate fluid intake, typically consumed as the athlete is sailing back to shore

- **More than 2 hours after competition:** A balance of carbohydrate and protein, with lower amounts of healthy fat and limited alcohol intake

BIBLIOGRAPHY

Chapter 1

Benardot, D., Martin, D., Thompson, W., and Roman, S. 2005. Between-meal energy intake affects body composition, performance and total caloric consumption in athletes. *Medicine and Science in Sports and Exercise* 37:S339.

Bompa, T. 1999. The basis for training. In *Periodization: Theory and methodology of training*. Edited by T. Bompa. Champaign, IL: Human Kinetics.

Bompa, T., and Omar., Y. 1999. Rest and recovery. In *Periodization: Theory and methodology of training*. Edited by T. Bompa. Champaign, IL: Human Kinetics.

Bullough, R., Gillette, C., Harris, M., and Melby, C. 1995. Interaction of acute changes in exercise energy expenditure and energy intake on resting metabolic rate. *American Journal of Clinical Nutrition* 61:473-481.

Burke, L., Collier, G., and Hargreaves, M. 1993. Muscle glycogen storage after prolonged exercise: The effect of glycemic index of carbohydrate feedings. *Journal of Applied Physiology* 75:1019-1023.

DeBock, K., Derave, W., Eijnde, B., Hesselink, M., Koninckx, E., Rose, A., Schrauwen, P., Bonen, A., Richter, E., and Hespel, P. 2008. Effect of training in the fasted state on metabolic responses during exercise with carbohydrate intake. *Journal of Applied Physiology* 104:1045-1055.

Deutz, B., Benardot, D., Martin, D., and Cody, M. 2000. Relationship between energy deficits and body composition in elite female gymnasts and runners. *Medicine and Science in Sports and Exercise* 32:659-668.

Ivy, J., Goforth, H., Damon, B., McCauley, T., Parsons, E., and Price, T. 2002. Early postexercise muscle glycogen recovery is enhanced with carbohydrate–protein supplement. *Journal of Applied Physiology* 93:1337-1344.

Ivy, J., Katz, A., Cutler, C., Sherman, W., and Coyle, E. 1988. Muscle glycogen synthesis after exercise: Effect of time of carbohydrate ingestions. *Journal of Applied Physiology* 64:1480-1485.

Iwao, S., Mori, K., and Sato, Y. 1996. Effects of meal frequency on body composition during weight control in boxers. *Scandinavian Journal of Medicine and Science in Sports* 6:265-272.

Noakes, T., Peltonen, J., and Rusko, H. 2001. Evidence that a central governor regulates exercise performance during acute hypoxia and hyperoxia. *Journal of Experimental Biology* 204:3225-3234.

Steen, S., Opplinger, R., and Brownell, K. 1988. Metabolic effects of repeated weight loss and regain in adolescent wrestlers. *Journal of the American Medical Association* 260:47-50.

Woods, S., and Seeley, R. 2000. Adiposity signals and the control of energy homeostasis. *Nutrition* 16:894-902.

Chapter 2

Ainsworth, B., Haskell, W., Leon, A., Jacobs, D., Montoye, H., Sallis, J., and Paffenbarger, R. 1993. Compendium of physical activities: Classification of energy costs of human physical activities. *Medicine and Science in Sports and Exercise* 25:71-80.

Foster, C., Florhaug, J., Franklin, J., Gottschall, L., Hrovatin, L., Parker, S., Doleshal, P., and Dodge, C. 2001. A new approach to monitoring exercise training. *Journal of Strength and Conditioning Research* 15:109-115.

Lacour, J., Bouvat, E., and Barthelemy, J. 1990. Post-competition blood lactate concentrations as indicators of anaerobic energy expenditure during 400-m and 800-m races. *European Journal of Applied Physiology* 61:172-176.

Meeusen, R., and De Meirleir, K. 1995. Exercise and brain neurotransmission. *Sports Medicine* 20:160-188.

Prochaska, J., and DiClemente, C. 1982. Transtheoretical therapy: Toward a more integrative model of change. *Psychotherapy: Theory, Research and Practice* 19:276-288.

Stubbs, R., van Wyk, M., Johnstone, A., and Harbron, C. 1996. Breakfasts high in protein, fat or carbohydrate: Effect on within-day appetite and energy balance. *European Journal of Clinical Nutrition* 50:409-417.

Chapter 3

Greene, G.W., Rossi, S.R., Rossi, J.S., Velicher, W.F., Fava, J.L., and Prochaska, J.O. 1999. Dietary applications of the stages of change model. *Journal of the American Dietetic Association* 99:673-678.

Sandoval, W.M., Heller, K.E., Wiese, W.H., and Childs, D.A. 1994. Stages of change: A model for nutrition counseling. *Topics in Clinical Nutrition* 9(3):64-69.

Chapter 4

Abbott, W., Howard, B., Christin, L., Freymond, D., Lillioja, S., Boyce, V., Anderson, T., Bogardus, C., and Ravussin, E. 1988. Short-term energy balance: Relationship with protein, carbohydrate and fat balances. *American Journal of Physiology* 255:E332-337.

Balsom, P., Wood, K., Olsson, P., and Ekblom, B. 1999. Carbohydrate intake and multiple sprint sports: With special reference to football (soccer). *International Journal of Sports Medicine* 13:152-157.

Bucci, L. 1993. *Nutrients as ergogenic aids for sports and exercise.* Boca Raton, FL: CRC Press.

Owasoyo, J., Neri, D., and Lamberth, J. 1992. Tyrosine and its potential use as a countermeasure to performance decrement in military sustained operations. *Aviation, Space, and Environmental Medicine* 63:364-369.

Palou, A., Pico, C., and Bonet, M. 2004. Food safety and functional foods in the European union: Obesity as a paradigmatic example for novel food development. *Nutrition Reviews* 62:S169-S181.

Thomas, C., Peters, J., Reed, G., Abumrad, N., Sun, M., and Hill, J. 1992. Nutrient balance and energy expenditure during ad libitum feeding of high-fat and high-carbohydrate diets in humans. *American Journal of Clinical Nutrition* 55:934-942.

Tipton, K., Elliott, T., Cree, M., Wolf, S., Sanford, A., and Wolfe, R. 2004. Ingestion of casein and whey proteins results in muscle anabolism after resistance exercise. *Medicine and Science in Sports and Exercise* 36:2073-2081.

Tipton, K., Rasmussen, B., Miller, S., Wolf, S., Owens-Stovall, S., Petrini, B., and Wolfe, R. 2001. Timing of amino acid-carbohydrate ingestion alters anabolic response of muscle to resistance exercise. *American Journal of Physiology* 281:E197-206.

Wallis, G., Dawson, R., Achten, J., Webber, J., and Jeukendrup, A. 2006. Metabolic response to carbohydrate ingestion during exercise in males and females. *American Journal of Physiology* 290: E708-715.

Chapter 5

Burke, L., and Deakin, V. 2006. *Clinical sports nutrition.* 3rd ed. Sydney: McGraw Hill Australia.

Cheuvront, S.N., Carter III, R., Montain, S.J., and Sawka, M.N. 2004. Daily body mass variability and stability in active men undergoing exercise-heat stress. *International Journal of Sport Nutrition and Exercise Metabolism* 14:532-540.

Cian, C., Koulmann, N., Barrand, P., Raphel, C., Jimenez, C., and Melin, B. 2000. Influence of variations in body hydration on cognitive function: Effect of hyperhydration, heat stress and exercise-induced dehydration. *Journal of Psychophysiology* 14:29-36.

Davis, J.M., and Bailey, S.P. 1997. Possible mechanisms of central nervous system fatigue during exercise. *Medicine and Science in Sports and Exercise* 29:45-57.

Dunford, M. 2006. *Sports nutrition: A practice manual for professionals.* Chicago: American Dietetic Association.

Dunford, M., and Doyle, J.A. 2008. *Nutrition for sport and exercise.* Belmont, CA: Thompson Higher Education.

Epstein, Y., Keren, G., Moisseiev, J., Gasko, O., and Yachin, S. 1980. Psychomotor deterioration during exposure to heat. *Aviation, Space, and Environmental Medicine* 51(6):607-610.

Gopinathan, P.M., Pichan, G., and Shanna, V.M. 1988. Role of dehydration in heat stress-induced variations in mental performance. *Archives of Environmental Health* 43:15-17.

Greenwood, M., Kreider, R.B., Greenwood, L., and Byars, A. 2003. Cramping and injury incidence in collegiate football players are reduced by creatine supplementation. *Journal of Athletic Training* 38:216-219.

Institute of Medicine. 2005. Water. In *Dietary reference intakes for water, sodium, chloride, potassium and sulfate*. Washington, DC: National Academies Press.

Jones, L.C., Cleary, M.A., Lopez, R.M., Zuri, R.E., and Lopez, R. 2008. Active dehydration impairs upper and lower body anaerobic muscular power. *Journal of Strength and Conditioning Research* 22(2):455-463.

Jung, A.P., Bishop, P.A., Al-Nawwa, A., and Dale, R.B. 2005. Influence of hydration and electrolyte supplementation on incidence and time to onset of exercise-associated muscle cramps. *Journal of Athletic Training* 40(2):71-75.

Kantorowski, P.B., Hiller, W.D.B., Garrett, W.E., Douglas, P.S., Smith, R., and O'Toole, M. 1990. Cramping studies in 2600 endurance athletes. *Medicine and Science in Sports and Exercise* 22(2):S104.

Kenney, W.L., Tankersley, C.G., Newswanger, D.L., Hyde, D.E., Puhl, S.M., and Turner, S.L. 1990. Age and hypohydration independently influence the peripheral vascular system response to heat stress. *Journal of Applied Physiology* 68:1902-1908.

Laursen, P.B., Suriano, R., Quod, M.J., Lee, H., Abbiss, C.R., Nosaka, K., Martin, D.T., and Bishop, D. 2006. Core temperature and hydration status during an Ironman triathlon. *British Journal of Sports Medicine* 40:320-325.

Maughan, R. 1986. Exercise induced muscle cramps: A prospective biochemical study in marathon runners. *Journal of Sports Sciences* 4:31-34.

Maughan, R., and Shirreffs, S.M. 2008. Development of individual hydration strategies for athletes. *International Journal of Sport Nutrition and Exercise Metabolism* 18:457-472.

Meyer, F., Bar-Or, O., MacDougall, J.D., and Heigenhauser, J.F. 1992. Sweat electrolyte loss during exercise in the heat: Effects of gender and maturation. *Medicine and Science in Sports and Exercise* 24:776-781.

Miles, M.P., and Clarkson, P.M. 1994. Exercise induced muscle pain, soreness and cramps. *Journal of Sports Medicine and Physical Fitness* 34:203-216.

Sawka, M.N., Burke, L.M., Eichner, E.R., Maughan, R.J., Montain, S.J., and Stachenfeld, N.S. 2007. Exercise and fluid replacement position stand. *Medicine and Science in Sports and Exercise* 39:377-389.

Sawka, M.N., and Pandolf, K.B. 1990. Effects of body water loss in physiological function and exercise performance. In *Perspectives in exercise science and sports medicine: Fluid homeostasis during exercise*. Edited by D.R. Lamb and C.V. Gisolfi. Indianapolis: Benchmark Press.

Sawka, M.N., Wenger, C.B., and Pandolf, K.B. 1996. Thermoregulatory responses to acute exercise-heat stress and heat acclimation. In *Handbook of physiology, section 4: Environmental physiology*. Edited by C.M. Blatteis and M.J. Fregly. New York: Oxford University Press.

Schwellnus, M.P., Derman, E.W., and Noakes, T.D. 1997. Aetiology of skeletal muscle "cramps" during exercise: A novel hypothesis. *Journal of Sports Science* 15:277-285.

Seckl, J.R., Williams, T.D.M., and Lightman, S.L. 1986. Oral hypertonic saline causes transient fall of vasopressin in humans. *American Journal of Physiology* 251:R214-R217.

Speedy, D.B., Noakes, T.D., and Schneider, C. 2001. Exercise-associated hyponatremia: A review. *Emergency Medicine* 13:17-27.

Thompson, C.J., Burd, J., and Baylis, P.H. 1987. Acute suppression of plasma vasopressin and thirst after drinking in hypernatremic humans. *American Journal of Physiology* 240:R1138-1142.

Williamson, S.L., Johnson, R.W., Hudkins, P.G., and Strate, S.M. 1993. Exertion cramps: A prospective study of biochemical and anthropometric variables in bicycle riders. *Cycling Science* Spring:15-20.

Chapter 6

Acheson, K.J., Schutz, Y., Bessard, T., Anantharaman, K., Flatt, J.P., and Jequier. 1988. Glycogen storage capacity and de novo lipogenesis during massive carbohydrate feeding in man. *American Journal of Clinical Nutrition* 48:240-247.

Bergstrom, J., Hermansen, L., Hultman, E., and Saltin, B. 1967. Diet, muscle glycogen and physical performance. *Acta Physiologica Scandinavica* 71:140-150.

Broad, E.M., Burke, L.M., Gox, G.R., Heeley, P., and Riley, M. 1996. Body weight changes and voluntary fluid intakes during training and competition sessions in team sports. *International Journal of Sport Nutrition* 6:307-320.

Bucci, L. 1993. *Nutrients as ergogenic aids for sports and exercise.* Boca Raton, FL: CRC Press.

Burke, L., Collier, G., and Hargreaves, M. 1993. Muscle glycogen storage after prolonged exercise: The effect of glycemic index of carbohydrate feedings. *Journal of Applied Physiology* 75:1019-1023.

Burke, L., and Deakin, V. 2006. *Clinical sports nutrition.* 3rd ed. Sydney: McGraw Hill Australia.

Burke, L.M., Collier, R., Beasley, S.K., Davis, P.G., Fricker, P.A., Heeley, P., Walder, K., and Hargreaves, M. 1995. Effect of coingestion of fat and protein with carbohydrate feedings on muscle glycogen storage. *Journal of Applied Physiology* 87:2187-2192.

Burke, L.M., Kiens, B., and Ivy, J.L. 2004. Carbohydrates and fat for training and recovery. *Journal of Sports Sciences* 22:15-30.

Costa, R.J., Jones, G.E., Lamb, K.L., Coleman, R., and Williams, J.H. 2005. The effects of a high carbohydrate diet on cortisol and salivary immunoglobin A (s-IgA) during a period of increased exercise workload amongst Olympic and Ironman triathletes. *International Journal of Sports Medicine* 26(10):880-885.

Costill, D.L., Pascoe, D.D., Fink, W.J., Robergs, R.A., Barr, S.I., and Pearson, D. 1990. Impaired muscle glycogen resynthesis after eccentric exercise. *Journal of Applied Physiology* 69:46-50.

Currell, K., and Jeukendrup, A.E. 2008. Superior endurance performance with ingestion of multiple transportable carbohydrates. *Medicine and Science in Sports and Exercise* 40(2):275-281.

DeBock, K., Derave, W., Eijnde, B., Hesselink, M., Koninckx, E., Rose, A., Schrauwen, P., Bonen, A., Richter, E., and Hespel, P. 2008. Effect of training in the fasted state on metabolic responses during exercise with carbohydrate intake. *Journal of Applied Physiology* 104:1045-1055.

Goedecke, J.H., Christie, C., Wilson, G., Dennis, S.C., Noakes, T.D., Hopkins, W.G., and Lambert, E.V. 1999. Metabolic adaptations to a high-fat diet in endurance cyclists. *Metabolism* 48:1509-1517.

Hawley, J.A., Schabort, E.J., Noakes, T.D., and Dennis, S.C. 1997. Carbohdyrate-loading and exercise performance: An update. *Sports Medicine* 24:73-81.

Ivy, J., Goforth, H., Damon, B., McCauley, T., Parsons, E., and Price, T. 2002. Early postexercise muscle glycogen recovery is enhanced with carbohydrate-protein supplement. *Journal of Applied Physiology* 93:1337-1344.

Ivy, J., Katz, A., Cutler, C., Sherman, W., and Coyle, E. 1988. Muscle glycogen synthesis after exercise: Effect of time of carbohydrate ingestions. *Journal of Applied Physiology* 64:1480-1485.

Jeukendrup, A.E., Saris, W.H., Brouns, F., Halliday, D., and Wagenmakers, A.J.M. 1996. Effects of carbohydrate and fat supplementation on CHO metabolism during prolonged exercise. *Metabolism* 46:915-921.

Jeukendrup, A.E., Saris, W.H.M., Schrauwen, P., Brouns, F., and Wagenmakers, A.J.M. 1995. Metabolic availability of medium-chain triglycerides coingested with carbohydrate during prolonged exercise. *Journal of Applied Physiology* 79:756-762.

Lambert, E.V., Hawley, J.A., Goedecke, J., Noakes, T.D., and Dennis, S.C. 1997. Nutritional strategies for promoting fat utilization and delaying the onset of fatigue during prolonged exercise. *Journal of Sports Sciences* 15:315-324.

Lopez-Garcia, E., Schulze, M.B., Manson, J.E., Meigs, J.B., Albert, C.M., Rifai, N., Willett, W.C., and Hu, F.B. 2004. Consumption of n-3 fatty acids is related to plasma biomarkers of inflammation and endothelial activation in women. *Journal of Nutrition* 134:1806-1811.

MacRae, H.S., Toakes, T.D., and Dennis, S.C. 1995. Role of decreased carbohydrate oxidation on slower rises in ventilation with increasing exercise intensity after training. *European Journal of Applied Physiology* 71:523-529.

Maughan, R.J., Leiper, J.B., and Shirreffs, S.M. 1996. Restoration of fluid balance after exercise-induced dehydration: Effects of food and fluid intake. *European Journal of Applied Physiology* 73:317-325.

Meeusen, R., and De Meirleir, K. 1995. Exercise and brain neurotransmission. *Sports Medicine* 20:160-188.

Mozaffarian, D., Pischon, T., Hankinson, S.E., Rifai, N., Joshipura, K., Willett, W.C., and Rimm, E.B. 2004. Dietary intake of trans fatty acids and systemic inflammation in women. *American Journal of Clinical Nutrition* 79:606-612.

Mujika, I., and Padilla, S. 2000. Detraining: Loss of training-induced physiological and performance adaptations. Part I: Short term insufficient training stimulus. *Sports Medicine* 30:79-87.

Newsholme, E.A., and Leech, A.R. 1983. *Biochemistry for the medical sciences.* Chichester: Wiley.

Nieman, D.C., and Pedersen, B.K. 1999. Exercise and immune function: Recent developments. *Sports Medicine* 27:73-80.

Noakes, T.D., Adams, B.A., Myburgh, K.H., Greff, C., Lotz, T., and Nathan, M. 1988. The danger of inadequate water intake during prolonged exercise. *European Journal of Applied Physiology* 57:10-19.

Simopoulos, A.P. 2007. Omega-3 fatty acids and athletics. *Current Sports Medicine Reports* 6:230-236.

Tipton, K., Elliott, T., Cree, M., Wolf, S., Sanford, A., and Wolfe, R. 2004. Ingestion of casein and whey proteins results in muscle anabolism after resistance exercise. *Medicine and Science in Sports and Exercise* 36:2073-2081.

Tipton, K., Rasmussen, B., Miller, S., Wolf, S., Owens-Stovall, S., Petrini, B., and Wolfe, R. 2001. Timing of amino acid–carbohydrate ingestion alters anabolic response of muscle to resistance exercise. *American Journal of Physiology* 281:E197-206.

VanLoon, L.J., Schrauwen-Hinderling, V.B., Koopman, R., Wagenmakers, A.J., Hesselink, M.K., Schart, G., Looi, M.E., and Saris, W.H. 2003. Influence of prolonged cycling and recovery diet on intramuscular triglyceride content in trained males. *American Journal of Physiology: Endocrinology and Metabolism* 285:E804-811.

Wallis, G., Dawson, R., Achten, J., Webber, J., and Jeukendrup, A. 2006. Metabolic response to carbohydrate ingestion during exercise in males and females. *American Journal of Physiology* 290:E708-715.

Walser, B., and Stebbins, C.L. 2008. Omega-3 fatty acid supplementation enhances stroke volume and cardiac output during dynamic exercise. *European Journal of Applied Physiology* 104:455-461.

Watt, M.J., Heigenhauser, G.J.F., and Spriet, L.L. 2002. Intramuscular triacylglycerol utilization in human skeletal muscle during exercise: Is there a controversy? *Journal of Applied Physiology* 93:1185-1195.

Chapter 7

Acheton, J., Gleeson, M., and Jeukendrup, A.E. 2002. Determination of the exercise intensity that elicits maximal fat oxidation. *Medicine and Science in Sports and Exercise* 34:92-97.

American Dietetic Association. 2003. Position of the American Dietetic Association and Dietitians of Canada: Vegetarian diets. *Journal of the American Dietetic Association* 103:748-765.

Burke, L.M., Collier, G.R., Beasley, S.K., Davis, P.G., Fricker, P.A., Heeley, P., Walder, K., and Hargreaves, M. 1995. Effect of coingestion of fat and protein with carbohydrate feedings on muscle glycogen storage. *Journal of Applied Physiology* 78:2187-2192.

Burke, L.M., Cox, G.R., Culmmings, N.K., and Desbrow, B. 2001. Guidelines for daily carbohydrate intake: Do athletes achieve them? *Sports Medicine* 31:267-299.

Burke, L.M., and Reed, R.S.D. 1987. Diet patterns of elite Australian male triathletes. *The Physician and Sportsmedicine* 15:140-155.

Butterfield, G. 1991. Amino acids and high protein diets. In *Perspectives in exercise science and sports medicine.* Edited by D. Lamb and M. Williams. Carmel, IN: Cooper.

Dohm, G.L., Beeker, R.T., Israel, R.G., and Tapscott, E.B. 1986. Metabolic response to exercise after fasting. *Journal of Applied Physiology* 61:1363-1368.

Eden, B.D., and Abernathy, P.J. 1994. Nutritional intake during an ultraendurance running race. *International Journal of Sport Nutrition* 4:166-174.

Gabel, K.A., Aldous, A., and Edgington, C. 1995. Dietary intake of two elite male cyclists during a 10-day, 2,050-mile ride. *International Journal of Sport Nutrition* 5:56-61.

Garcia-Roves, P.M., Terrados, N., Fernandez, S.F., and Patterson, A.M. 1998. Macronutrient intakes of top-level cyclists during continuous competition: Change in feeding pattern. *International Journal of Sports Medicine* 19:61-67.

Ivy, J.L., Lee, M.C., Broznick, J.T., and Reed, M.J. 1988. Muscle glycogen storage after different amounts of carbohydrate ingestion. *Journal of Applied Physiology* 65:2018-2023.

Laursen, P.B., and Rhodes, E.C. 1999. Physiological analysis of a high-intensity ultraendurance event. *Journal of Strength and Conditioning Research* 21:26-38.

Laursen, P.B., and Rhodes, E.C. 2000. Factors affecting performance in an ultraendurance triathlon. *Sports Medicine* 31:679-689.

Lindeman, A.K. Nutrient intake of an ultraendurance cyclist. 1991. *International Journal of Sport Nutrition* 1:79-85.

Rodriguez, N.R., DiMarco, N., and Langley, S. 2009. Position of the American Dietetic Association, Dietitians of Canada, and the American College of Sports Medicine: Nutrition and athletic performance. *Journal of Athletic Training* 109(3):509-527.

Saris, W.H.M., van Erp-Baart, M.A., Brouns, F., Westerterp, K.R., and ten Hoor, F. 1989. Study of food intake and energy expenditure during extreme sustained exercise: The Tour de France. *International Journal of Sports Medicine* 10(suppl):26-31.

Sports, Cardiovascular, and Wellness Nutritionists (SCAN). 2000. Carbohydrates and exercise. In *Sports nutrition: A guide for the professional working with active people*. Chicago: American Dietetic Association.

Tarnopolsky, M.A., Bosman, M., MacDonald, J.R., Vandeputte, D., Martin, J., and Roy, B.D. 1997. Postexercise protein-carbohydrate supplements increase muscle glycogen in men and women. *Journal of Applied Physiology* 83:1877-1883.

Chapter 8

American Dietetic Association. 2003. Position of the American Dietetic Association and Dietitians of Canada: Vegetarian diets. *Journal of the American Dietetic Association* 103:748-765.

Brown, E.C., DiSilvestro, R.A., Babaknia, A., and Devor, S.T. 2004. Soy versus whey protein bars: Effects on exercise training impact on lean body mass and antioxidant status. *Nutrition Journal* 3:1-5.

Burke, L., and Deakin, V. 2006. *Clinical sports nutrition*. 3rd ed. Sydney: McGraw Hill Australia.

Centers for Disease Control and Prevention. 2002. Iron deficiency: United States, 1999-2000. *Morbidity and Mortality Weekly Report* 51:897–899.

Crooks, C., Wall, C., Cross, M., and Rutherford-Markwick, K. 2006. The effect of bovine colostrum supplementation on salivary IgA in distance runners. *International Journal of Sport Nutrition and Exercise Metabolism* 16:47-64.

Deldicque, L., and Francaux, M. 2008. Functional food for exercise performance: Fact or foe? *Current Opinion in Clinical Nutrition and Metabolic Care* 11:774-781.

Driskell, J. 2006. Summary: Vitamins and trace elements in sports nutrition. In *Sports nutrition: Vitamins and trace elements*. Edited by J. Driskell and I. Wolinsky. New York: CRC/Taylor & Francis.

Easton, C., Turner, S., and Pitsiladis, Y. 2007. Creatine and glycerol hyperhydration in trained subjects before exercise in the heat. *International Journal of Sport Nutrition and Exercise Metabolism* 17:70-91.

Ganji, V., and Kies, C.V. 1996. Psyllium husk fiber supplementation to the diets rich in soybean or coconut oil: Hypocholesterolemic effect in healthy humans. *International Journal of Food Sciences and Nutrition* 47(2):103-110.

Hoffman, J.R., and Falvo, M.J. 2004. Protein: Which is best? *Journal of Science and Medicine in Sports* 3:118-130.

Institute of Medicine, Food and Nutrition Board. 2000. *Dietary reference intakes for thiamine, riboflavin, niacin, vitamin B_6, folate, vitamin B_{12}, pantothenic acid, biotin and choline*. Washington, DC: National Academies Press.

Jenkins, D., Wolever, T., Rao, A.V., Hegele, R.A., Mitchell, S.J., Ransom, T., Boctor, D.L., Spadafora, P.J., Jenkins, A.L., Mehling, C., Katzman Relle, L., Connelly, P.W., Story, J.A., Furumoto, E.J., Corey, P., and Wursch, P. 1993. Effect on blood lipids of very high intakes of fiber in diets low in saturated fat and cholesterol. *New England Journal of Medicine* 329:21-26.

Jenkinson, D., and Harbert, A. 2008. Supplements and sports. *American Family Physician* 78:1039-46.

Khan, F., Elherik, K., Bolton-Smith, C., Barr, R., Hill, A., Murrie, I., and Belch, J.J. 2003. The effects of dietary fatty acid supplementation on endothelial function and vascular tone in healthy subjects. *Cardiovascular Research* 59(4):955-962.

Lukaski, H.C. 2004. Vitamin and mineral status: Effects on physical performance. *Nutrition* 20:632-644.

Magkos, F., and Kavouras, S. 2005. Caffeine use in sports, pharmacokinetics in man, and cellular mechanisms of action. *Critical Reviews in Food Science and Nutrition* 45:535-62.

Maughan, R.J., Depiesse, F., and Geyer, H. 2007. The use of dietary supplements by athletes. *Journal of Sports Sciences* 25:S103-113.

McNaughton, L., Siegler, J., and Midgley, A. 2008. Ergogenic effects of sodium bicarbonate. *Current Sports Medicine Reports* 7(4):230-236.

Mickelborough, T.D., Murray, R.L., Ionescu, A.A., and Lindley, M.R. 2003. Fish oil supplementation reduces severity of exercise-induced bronchoconstriction in elite athletes. *American Journal of Respiratory and Critical Care Medicine* 168:1181-1189.

Monsen, E., Hallberg, L., Layrisse, M., Hegsted, D., Cook, J., Mertz, W., and Finch, C. 1978. Estimation of available dietary iron. *American Journal of Clinical Nutrition* 31:134-141

Montner, P., Stark, D., Riedesel, M., Murata, G., Robergs, R., Timms, M., and Chick, T. 1996. Pre-exercise glycerol hydration improves cycling endurance time. *International Journal of Sports Medicine* 17:27-33.

Nattiv, A., Loucks, A., Manore, M., Sanborn, C., Sundgot-Borgen, J., and Warren, M. 2007. American College of Sports Medicine position stand: The female athlete triad. *Medicine and Science in Sports and Exercise* 39:1867-1882.

Phillips, S.M., Moore, D.R., and Tang, J.E. 2007. A critical examination of dietary protein requirements, benefits and excesses in athletes. *International Journal of Sport Nutrition and Exercise Metabolism* 17:S58-76.

Powers, S.K., DeRuisseau, K.C., Quindry, J., and Hamilton, K.L. 2004. Dietary antioxidants and exercise. *Journal of Sports Science* 22:81-94.

Queenan, K.M., Stewart, M.L., Smith, K.N., Thomas, W., Fulcher, R.G., and Slavin, J.L. 2007. Concentrated oat beta-glucan, a fermentable fiber, lowers serum cholesterol in hypercholesterolemic adults in a randomized controlled trial. *Nutrition Journal* 6:1-8.

Rodriguez, N.R., DiMarco, N., and Langley, S. 2009. Position of the American Dietetic Association, Dietitians of Canada, and the American College of Sports Medicine: Nutrition and athletic performance. *Journal of the American Dietetic Association* 109(3):509-527.

Shing, C., Peake, J., Suzuki, K., Okutsu, M., Pereira, R., Stevenson, L., Jenkins, D., and Coombes, J. 2007. Effects of bovine colostrum supplementation on immune variables in highly trained cyclists. *Journal of Applied Physiology* 102:1113-1122.

Simopoulos, A.P. 2007. Omega-3 fatty acids and athletics. *Current Sports Medicine Reports* 6:230-236.

Tipton, K.D., Elliott, T.A., Cree, M.G., Aarsland, A.A., Sanford, A.P., and Wolfe, R.R. 2007. Stimulation of net muscle protein synthesis by whey protein ingestion before and after exercise. *American Journal of Physiology: Endocrinology and Metabolism* 292:E71-76.

Tremblay, M., Galloway, S., and Sexsmith, J. 1994. Ergogenic effects of phosphate loading: Physiological fact or methodological fiction. *Canadian Journal of Applied Physiology* 19:1-11.

Vellar, O. 1968. Studies on sweat losses of nutrients. I. Iron content of whole body sweat and its association with other sweat constituents, serum iron levels, hematological indices, body surface area, and sweat rate. *Scandinavian Journal of Clinical Investigation* 21:157-167.

Walser, B., Giordano, R.M., and Stebbins, C.L. 2006. Supplementation with omega-3 polyunsaturated fatty acids augments brachial artery dilation and blood flow during forearm contraction. *European Journal of Applied Physiology* 97:347-354.

Walser, B., and Stebbins, C.L. 2008. Omega-3 fatty acid supplementation enhances stroke volume and cardiac output during dynamic exercise. *European Journal of Applied Physiology* 104:455-461.

Watson, T.A., Callister, R., Taylor, R.D., Sibbritt, D.W., MacDonald-Wicks, L.K., and Garg, M.L. 2005. Antioxidant restriction and oxidative stress in short-duration exhaustive exercise. *Medicine and Science in Sports and Exercise* 37:63-71.

Wilkinson, S.B., Tarnopolsky, M.A., MacDonald, M.J., MacDonald, J.R., Armstrong,

D., and Phillips, S.M. 2007. Consumption of fluid skim milk promotes greater muscle protein accretion after resistance exercise than does consumption of isonitrogenous and isoenergetic soy-protein beverage. *American Journal of Clinical Nutrition* 85(4):1031-1040.

Williams, S.L., Strobel, M.A., Lexis, L.A., and Coombes, J.S. 2006. Antioxidant requirements of endurance athletes: Implications for health. *Nutrition Reviews* 64(3):93-108.

Woolf, K., and Manore, M.M. 2006. B-vitamins and exercise: Does exercise alter requirements? *International Journal of Sports Nutrition and Exercise Metabolism* 16:453-484.

Chapter 9

Armstrong, L., Hubbard, R., Askew, E., De Luca, J., O'Brien, C., Pasqualicchio, A., and Francesconi, R. 1993. Responses to moderate and low sodium diets during exercise–heat acclimation. *International Journal of Sport Nutrition* 3:207-221.

Florida-James, G., Donaldson, K., Stone, V. 2004. Athens 2004: The pollution climate and athletic performance. *Journal of Sport Sciences* 22:967-980.

Mickleborough, T., Lindley, M., Ionescu, A., and Fly, A. 2006. Protective effect of fish oil supplementation on exercise-induced bronchoconstriction in asthma. *Chest* 129:39-49.

Montain, S. 2008. Hydration recommendations for sport. *Current Sports Medicine Reports* 7:187-192.

Pandolf, K., Sawka, M., and Gonzalez, R. eds. 1988. *Human performance physiology and environmental medicine at terrestrial extremes.* Indianapolis: Benchmark Press.

Chapter 10

Costill, D., Cote, R., and Fink, W. 1976. Muscle water and electrolytes following varied levels of dehydration in man. *Journal of Applied Physiology* 40:6-11.

Ivy, J. 2004. Regulation of muscle glycogen repletion, muscle protein synthesis and repair following exercise. *Journal of Sports Science and Medicine* 3:131-138.

Lieberman, H., Caruso, C., Niro, P., Adam, G., Kellogg, M., Nindl, B., and Kramer, M. 2008. A double-blind, placebo controlled test of 2 d of calorie deprivation: Effects on cognition, activity, sleep and interstitial glucose concentrations. *American Journal of Clinical Nutrition* 88:667-676.

Nindl, B., Leone, C., Tharion, W., Johnson, R., Casellani, J., Patton, J., and Montain, S. 2002. Physical performance responses during 72 h of military operational stress. *Medicine and Science in Sports and Exercise* 34:1814-1822.

Rankin, J., Ocel, J., and Craft, L. 1996. Effect of weight loss and refeeding diet composition on anaerobic performance in wrestlers. *Medicine and Science in Sports and Exercise* 28:1292-1299.

Slater, G., Rice, A., Sharpe, K., Jenkins, D., and Hahn, A. 2007. Influence of nutrient intake after weigh-in on lightweight rowing performance. *Medicine and Science in Sports and Exercise* 39:184-191.

Tarnopolsky, M., Cipriano, N., Woodcroft, C., Pulkkinen, W., Robinson, D., Henderson, J., and MacDougall, J. 1996. Effects of rapid weight loss and wrestling on muscle glycogen concentration. *Clinical Journal of Sport Medicine* 6:78-84.

INDEX

Note: The italicized *f* and *t* following page numbers refer to figures and tables, respectively.

ABOUT THE AUTHORS

Krista Austin, PhD, CSCS, is an exercise physiologist, nutritionist, and NSCA-certified strength and conditioning specialist. She is also a research associate with the International Center for East African Running Studies.

Austin was a performance nutritionist with the English Institute of Sport, where she provided services to 18 Olympic sports and the England cricket team. Most recently she served as a physiologist with the United States Olympic Committee, where she worked with multiple sports in preparation for the 2008 Olympic Games. In particular, she is well known for her nutrition work with USA Taekwondo.

Austin is owner of Performance & Nutrition Coaching, LLC, which provides physiological testing, nutrition, and coaching education to professional and amateur athletes as well as Olympic national teams, including athletes competing for USA Track & Field, USA Canoe/Kayak, USA Wrestling, and USA Triathlon.

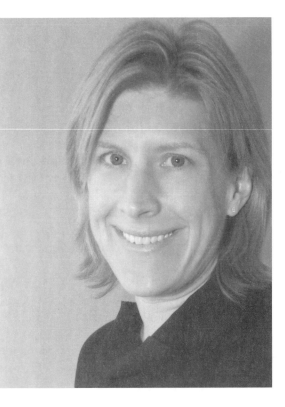

A former collegiate tennis player, she obtained a PhD in movement science from Florida State University and holds a master's degree in exercise physiology from San Diego State University. She is a member of the American College of Sports Medicine and has also served as associate editor of the *International Journal of Sport Nutrition and Exercise Metabolism*.

Bob Seebohar, MS, RD, CSSD, CSCS, is a board-certified specialist in sport dietetics and owner of Fuel4mance, a leading nutrition consulting firm serving amateur and elite athletes. Seebohar is the former director of sport nutrition for the University of Florida and most recently served as a sport dietitian for the U.S. Olympic Committee. In 2008, Seebohar traveled to the Summer Olympic Games in Beijing as a sport dietitian for the U.S. Olympic team and as the personal sport dietitian for the Olympic triathlon team. Seebohar currently consults as a sport dietitian for US Sailing (Olympic and Paralympic sailors) and the USA Triathlon national athletes and 2012 and 2016 Olympic team athletes.

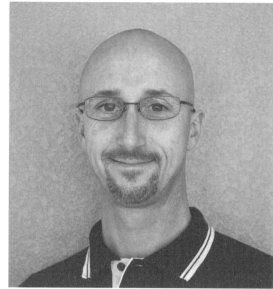

Seebohar has worked with athletes in a variety of sports, including triathlon, duathlon, ultrarunning and cycling, track and field, marathon, mountain biking, road and track cycling, cross country, swimming, football, taekwondo, motocross, tennis, wrestling, weightlifting, rowing, sailing, canoeing, and kayaking. He has worked with people of all ages and abilities, including high school students, recreationally active adults, professional athletes, and Olympians.

Seebohar holds a bachelor's degree in exercise and sport science and master's degrees in health and exercise science and food science and human nutrition. He is a registered dietitian, exercise physiologist, certified strength and conditioning specialist, and a high-performance triathlon coach.

Beginning as a competitive soccer player in his youth, Seebohar turned to endurance sports in 1993. In 1996 he represented the United States as a member of the 1996 duathlon team at the 1996 World Championships. He has competed in numerous endurance events, including the Boston Marathon, six Ironman races, the Leadville 100-mile trail race, and the Leadville 100-mile mountain bike race. In 2009, Seebohar became a Leadman, completing all six of the Leadville endurance events in seven weeks.

He lives in Littleton, Colorado, where he enjoys training for ultraendurance running and cycling events and coaching youth in soccer and triathlon.